The Equine Foot: Moving the Needle to Best Care

Editor

JAMES A. ORSINI

VETERINARY CLINICS OF NORTH AMERICA: EQUINE PRACTICE

www.vetequine.theclinics.com

Consulting Editor
THOMAS J. DIVERS

December 2021 • Volume 37 • Number 3

ELSEVIER

1600 John F. Kennedy Boulevard ● Suite 1800 ● Philadelphia, Pennsylvania, 19103-2899

http://www.vetequine.theclinics.com

VETERINARY CLINICS OF NORTH AMERICA: EQUINE PRACTICE Volume 37, Number 3
December 2021 ISSN 0749-0739, ISBN-13: 978-0-323-96081-6

Editor: Katerina Heidhausen
Developmental Editor: Ann Gielou Posedio

Veterinary Clinics of North America: Equine Practice (ISSN 0749-0739) is published in April, August, and December by Elsevier Inc., 360 Park Avenue South, New York, NY 10010-1710. Business and Editorial Offices: 1600 John F. Kennedy Blvd., Suite 1800, Philadelphia, PA 19103-2899. Subscription prices are $293.00 per year (domestic individuals), $766.00 per year (domestic institutions), $100.00 per year (domestic students/residents), $334.00 per year (Canadian individuals), $820.00 per year (Canadian institutions), $365.00 per year (international individuals), $820.00 per year (international institutions), $100.00 per year (Canadian students/residents), and $180.00 per year (international students/residents). To receive student/resident rate, orders must be accompanied by name of affiliated institution, date of term, and the signature of program/residency coordinator on institution letterhead. Orders will be billed at individual rate until proof of status is received. Foreign air speed delivery is included in all *Clinics* subscription prices. All prices are subject to change without notice. **POSTMASTER:** Send address changes to *Veterinary Clinics of North America: Equine Practice*, 3251 Riverport Lane, Maryland Heights, MO 63043. Customer Service (orders, claims, online, change of address): Elsevier Health Sciences Division, Subscription **Customer Service, 3251 Riverport Lane, Maryland Heights, MO 63043. Tel: 1-800-654-2452 (U.S. and Canada); 314-447-8871 (outside U.S. and Canada). Fax: 314-447-8029. E-mail: journalscustomerservice-usa@elsevier.com (for print support);** E-mail: **journalsonlinesupport-usa@ elsevier.com (for online support).**

Reprints. For copies of 100 or more of articles in this publication, please contact the Commercial Reprints Department, Elsevier Inc., 360 Park Avenue South, New York, NY 10010-1710. Tel.: 212-633-3874; Fax: 212-633-3820; E-mail: reprints@elsevier.com.

Veterinary Clinics of North America: Equine Practice is covered in *MEDLINE/PubMed (Index Medicus), Excerpta Medica, Current Contents/Agriculture, Biology and Environmental Sciences,* and *ISI.*

Contributors

CONSULTING EDITOR

THOMAS J. DIVERS, DVM

Diplomate, American College of Veterinary Internal Medicine; Diplomate, American College of Veterinary Emergency and Critical Care; Steffen Professor of Veterinary Medicine, Department of Clinical Sciences, Section of Large Animal Medicine, College of Veterinary Medicine, Cornell University, Ithaca, New York, USA

EDITOR

JAMES A. ORSINI, DVM

Diplomate, American College of Veterinary Surgeons; Associate Professor of Surgery, Department of Clinical Studies, New Bolton Center, University of Pennsylvania School of Veterinary Medicine, Kennett Square, Pennsylvania, USA

AUTHORS

RAUL BRAS, DVM, CJF

Part of the Division/Section of Equine Podiatry, Rood & Riddle Equine Hospital, Lexington, Kentucky, USA

TERESA A. BURNS, DVM, PhD

Diplomate, American College of Veterinary Internal Medicine; Associate Professor, Equine Internal Medicine, Department of Veterinary Clinical Sciences, The Ohio State University, Columbus, Ohio, USA

BERND DRIESSEN, DVM, PhD, Dipl ACVAA

Diplomate, European College of Veterinary Pharmacology and Toxicology; Department of Clinical Studies, School of Veterinary Medicine, University of Pennsylvania, Kennett Square, Pennsylvania, USA

JULIE ENGILES, BA, VMD

Diplomate, American College of Veterinary Pathology; Associate Professor of Pathology, Department of Clinical Studies, New Bolton Center, School of Veterinary Medicine, University of Pennsylvania, Kennett Square, Pennsylvania, USA

LEE ANN FUGLER, DVM, PhD

Department of Veterinary Clinical Sciences, Louisiana State University, School of Veterinary Medicine, Baton Rouge, Louisiana, USA

ANTON E. FÜRST, Dr med vet

Diplomate, European College of Veterinary Surgeons; Professor, Equine Department, Vetsuisse Faculty, University of Zurich, Zurich, Switzerland

HANNAH GALANTINO-HOMER, VMD, PhD
Diplomate, American College of Theriogenology; Senior Investigator in Laminitis Research, Department of Clinical Studies, New Bolton Center, School of Veterinary Medicine, University of Pennsylvania, Kennett Square, Pennsylvania, USA

AITOR GALLASTEGUI, LV, MSc
Diplomate, American College of Veterinary Radiology; Clinical Assistant Professor, Small Animal Clinical Sciences, University of Florida, Gainesville, Florida, USA

MATHEW P. GERARD, BVSc, PhD
Teaching Professor, Veterinary Anatomy, Department of Molecular Biomedical Sciences, North Carolina State University, College of Veterinary Medicine, Raleigh, North Carolina, USA

NORA S. GRENAGER, VMD
Diplomate, American College of Veterinary Internal Medicine (Large Animal); Medical Director, Steinbeck Peninsula Equine Clinics, Menlo Park, California, USA

KLAUS HOPSTER, PhD, DMV, DVM
Diplomate, European College of Veterinary Anaesthesia and Analgesia; Department of Clinical Studies, School of Veterinary Medicine, University of Pennsylvania, Kennett Square, Pennsylvania, USA

BRITTA SIGRID LEISE, DVM, PhD
Diplomate, American College of Veterinary Surgeons - Large Animal; Department of Veterinary Clinical Sciences, Louisiana State University, School of Veterinary Medicine, Baton Rouge, Louisiana, USA

CHRISTOPH J. LISCHER, Dr med vet
Diplomate, European College of Veterinary Surgeons; Professor, Faculty of Veterinary Medicine, Equine Clinic, Freie Universität Berlin, Berlin, Germany

DANIELA LUETHY, DVM
Diplomate, American College of Veterinary Internal Medicine - Large Animal Internal Medicine; Clinical Assistant Professor, Large Animal Medicine, Department of Large Animal Clinical Sciences, University of Florida, College of Veterinary Medicine, Gainesville, Florida, USA

SCOTT MORRISON, DVM
Head of Podiatry, Equine Podiatry, Rood & Riddle Equine Hospital, Lexington, Kentucky, USA

JAMES A. ORSINI, DVM
Diplomate, American College of Veterinary Surgeons; Associate Professor of Surgery, Department of Clinical Studies, New Bolton Center, University of Pennsylvania School of Veterinary Medicine, Kennett Square, Pennsylvania, USA

ANDREW VAN EPS, BVSc, PhD, MACVSc
Diplomate, American College of Veterinary Internal Medicine; Associate Professor, Department of Clinical Studies, New Bolton Center, School of Veterinary Medicine, University of Pennsylvania, Kennett Square, Pennsylvania, USA

Contents

New evidence suggests that a lack of limb load cycling activity (normally associated with ambulation) interferes with normal perfusion of the lamellae in these cases, resulting in ischemia and dysfunction/death of cells critical to the mechanical function of the lamellae. Excessive weight-bearing load drives the progression to overt acute laminitis in the supporting limb. Monitoring and enhancement of limb load cycling activity are key strategies that may lead to successful prevention of SLL by ensuring adequate lamellar perfusion.

Nutrition plays an important role in equine health, including that of the foot. Deficiencies and excesses of dietary components can affect the growth and function of the foot and have been associated with important podiatric diseases. The recognition, prevention, and treatment of specific notable nutritional diseases of the foot are discussed, as well as information regarding specific ingredients included in supplements meant to improve equine hoof quality. Ensuring provision of a balanced diet, maintaining horses in appropriate body condition, and seeking guidance from an equine nutritionist when creating dietary recommendations will prevent most equine foot disease related to nutrition.

Treatment of equine laminitis continues to be a challenge despite recent advancements in knowledge of the pathophysiology of laminitis. With more evidence supporting its use, distal limb hypothermia or cryotherapy has become a standard of care for both prevention of laminitis and treatment of the early stages of acute laminitis. Recent studies have demonstrated that cryotherapy reduces the severity of sepsis-related laminitis and hyperinsulinemic laminitis in experimental models and reduces the incidence of laminitis in clinical colitis cases. This article reviews the recent literature supporting the use of distal limb cryotherapy in horses.

Many disorders affect the equine foot, and many hoof problems have multiple predisposing causes. Surgery may be necessary after conservative management has failed. Diseases of the hoof capsule may seem simple, but their effect on performance can be long-lasting and healing is often prolonged. Diagnosis of problems within the hoof capsule is enhanced with the use of computed tomography and MRI. The prognosis of fractures has improved with strategic placement of lag screws across fracture planes using aiming devices and advanced intraoperative imaging techniques. Collaboration between the clinician and a skilled farrier is important for successful management of hoof disorders.

VETERINARY CLINICS OF NORTH AMERICA: EQUINE PRACTICE

RELATED SERIES

Veterinary Clinics of North America: Food Animal Practice
https://www.vetfood.theclinics.com/

THE CLINICS ARE NOW AVAILABLE ONLINE!
Access your subscription at:
www.theclinics.com

Preface

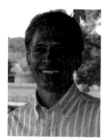

James A. Orsini, DVM
Editor

This issue of *Veterinary Clinics of North America: Equine Practice* builds on the foundation started in earlier issues of *Veterinary Clinics of North America: Equine Practice* that were topical on laminitis. This issue is an expanded and thoroughly updated issue that provides our fellow colleagues with a comprehensive and thorough resource for the "common" and "less common" problems of the equine foot and not just focused on laminitis. The information is the most exhaustive of any of the previous publications on the equine foot, while offering a point-by-point discussion of best practices when caring for the foot. Our goal, as a group, was to provide the most current, in-depth information for effectively managing the important clinical foot problems in the horse along with creating the framework in anatomy, physiology, pharmacology, nutrition, endocrinology, foot mechanics, and imaging, as well as recommendations and treatment options. The format is like other *Veterinary Clinics of North America: Equine Practice* issues and includes many illustrations, protocols, procedures, and treatments, clearly differentiating it from earlier publications on laminitis.

I recognize that there is more than one way to treat an equine foot problem, to diagnose a foot problem, or to perform a procedure, and to that extent this text is not a maxim but the compilation of experienced clinicians from both academia and private practice writing about these problems of the horse, and treatments in their area of expertise. There are 11 chapters, with every part the most current information on the topic and comprising feedback from our colleagues and friends who regularly treat the equine species.

Here are some of the highlights of this Veterinary Clinics of North America: Equine Practice issue:

- The first several chapters develop the important framework in anatomy, physiology, pain management, and imaging of the foot. I believe you will find the information comprehensive, covering the complex foot anatomy, consisting of multiple other interconnected systems: integument, musculoskeletal, nervous, and cardiovascular, as examples of the obvious groups. Appropriate management of the

Vet Clin Equine 37 (2021) ix–x
https://doi.org/10.1016/j.cveq.2021.09.002
0749-0739/21/© 2021 Published by Elsevier Inc.

pain associated with the pathology and mechanics of the foot is too commonly the one factor that tips the scale toward humane destruction, recognizing that foot pathology, and especially laminitis, with a rapid onset and a slow recovery, would have a better outcome if we could "buy the time" for therapeutic remediation.

- Tables and figures are included in this issue for a better understanding of the topic and to aid in illustrating key points.
- Imaging has taken on a whole new role now that we have adapted and perfected the technologies in computed tomography, MRI, nuclear scintigraphy (bone scans), ultrasonography, digital radiography, and more recently, PET. These imaging technologies have improved our abilities, as clinicians, to diagnose problems sooner, operate better, and improve treatment options and outcome by having a clearer diagnosis.
- There is an old saying among horsemen, "No foot, no horse." Horses are particularly delicate animals, considering their size and strength. Four willowy legs and various sized hooves that bear the horse's full weight of several hundred to over 1000 kg. The understanding of foot mechanics has made important advances with new materials, techniques, and preventive procedures that support the injured and diseased foot during healing.
- In addition to supporting the foot mechanically, we need to be sure we are feeding the foot for best health and "durability," understand the underlying causes for example, equine metabolic syndrome, SIRS, and support limb laminitis, and are prepared to prevent and treat the foot appropriately using "best"-in-class cryotherapy methods.
- And finally, recognizing the many foot problems affecting the horse that need to be considered in our differential diagnosis improves our ability to enhance the prognosis and make us better clinicians.

Thank you to my colleague and friend, Dr Tom Divers, Consulting Editor, for the invitation and opportunity to serve as the Guest Editor and contributing author for this issue of *Veterinary Clinics of North America: Equine Practice*, and to my colleagues and friends, who so generously afforded their time and expertise in advancing our understanding of the equine foot as contributing authors.

James A. Orsini, DVM
Department of Clinical Studies–
New Bolton Center
University of Pennsylvania
School of Veterinary Medicine
Kennett Square, PA 19348, USA

E-mail address:
Orsini@upenn.edu

The Big Picture in Better Understanding the Equine Foot

James A. Orsini, DVM

KEYWORDS

- Horse • Foot • Laminitis • Imaging • Pain management • Nutrition • Cryotherapy
- Foot mechanics

KEY POINTS

- Laminitis is an important disease of the equine foot.
- Multiple advances in imaging, for example, MRI, have helped in the diagnosis and treatment of foot diseases.
- Pain management using a multimodal approach has resulted in improved equine health care with foot diseases.
- Proper nutrition, cryotherapy, and good foot mechanics have advanced the care and welfare of the horse with foot problems.

INTRODUCTION

As I sit at my desk on this glorious day, the sun is glistening and inspires me to share my optimism and thoughts on the advances we have made in better understanding the equine foot.

Preparing the Introduction for this issue of the Veterinary Clinics of North America (VEP) - Equine (E) has filled me with gratitude to all those who generously contributed to its publication. The topics are comprehensive and in-depth, exploring concepts and describing experiences from many sources and clinicians. This new compilation includes state-of-the-art information on research that will transform clinical innovation for years to come.

The goal of this publication is to bring together participants and experts in all areas of equine care, to share information on better understanding the pathophysiology of foot diseases—encompassing prevention, research, and therapies for the many dreaded diseases of the foot and one at the forefront, laminitis!

The range and diversity of topics covered expanded geometrically as I planned this edition, with articles on feeding the foot, basic anatomy of the foot, and research with

Department of Clinical Studies – New Bolton Center, School of Veterinary Medicine, University of Pennsylvania, 382 West Street Road, Kennett Square, PA 19348, USA
E-mail address: orsini@upenn.edu

Vet Clin Equine 37 (2021) 521–528
https://doi.org/10.1016/j.cveq.2021.07.001
0749-0739/21/© 2021 Elsevier Inc. All rights reserved.

applications to the clinical setting. None of this would have been possible without the inspired help and contributions of many colleagues supporting the endeavor. As you read this edition of VEP, know that this is a collective effort of many dedicated faculty listed in the Table of Contents.

The common understanding of the foot from earlier issues of VEP provided a solid platform from which to expand and succeed in stimulating new interest in foot research and treatment. Increasing awareness of problems of the foot helped earlier diagnoses and treatment of affected horses.

LAMINITIS

The plight of famous racehorses—such as Secretariat, who, in 1973, captured the Thoroughbred Triple Crown and later succumbed to laminitis at the young age of 19 years, and most recently, Barbaro, in 2006—served to expand the general awareness of equine foot problems and laminitis specifically. For example, progress has been made in 3 specific, major areas of the laminitis battlefront:

1. Prevention progress: Widespread testing of horses at a younger age has shown that for equine metabolic syndrome and pars intermedia dysfunction, commonly known as equine Cushing disease, the use of medications and changes to nutrition thwarts the onset of laminitis.
2. Treatment progress: Innovative mechanical improvement in shoeing techniques and improved pain management technique have given us additional tools to provide horses under care a better quality of life.
3. Research progress: Increasing scientific data support the contention that the underlying pathophysiology of laminitis is an inflammatory process with secondary vascular complications, apart from support or contralateral laminitis where the vascular component likely comes first. These findings paved the way for many pharmaceutical advances.

As with any undertaking, it is important to understand where it began, the challenges faced, the current "situation," and long-term, future visions. Earlier publications in VEP addressed specific diseases of the equine foot, combining research and clinical approaches to solving multiple afflictions.

Although the progress has been great, we still have a long way to go. For instance, the goal of eradicating laminitis and other diseases of the foot has many similarities to medicine's approach to beating many human diseases. This goal is a complex endeavor that requires great patience, as well as endless hard work over an extended period.

As we pause to assess our current progress, we continually develop and refine our vision for the future. This seems to be the proper time to share that vision with the contributions of our colleagues who are experts in their disciplines. Our goal is to set precedents and establish methods of treatment and care to serve as the benchmark for veterinary care of the equine foot.

By expanding the base of "best-approach" knowledge, state-of-the art management of equine foot problems, and the destinctive anatomy, becomes more uniform throughout the equine community, and then limited treatment can be focused on the specific problems being treated.

In many ways, as commented on earlier, the efforts to manage difficult foot problems—for example, laminitis—parallels the war on cancer and heart disease, as 2 simple examples, which has been waged in human medicine for many decades. Many years ago, a diagnosis of cancer in humans was a death sentence. The diagnosis was a harbinger of a long, agonizing struggle almost certain to destroy a life and traumatize loved ones. The war against cancer has come a long way in the past several decades and, until recently, diagnoses of foot problems and laminitis were usually a death sentence for our equine friends.

Several specialties have improved our ability to better diagnose, prevent, manage, and treat diseases of the foot, including imaging, pain management, nutrition, cryotherapy, and farrier options for mechanical support of an unstable foot. These and many more topics of interest will be covered in this edition of VEP.

I'd like to review some of the important developments in each of these disciplines and how they relate to better "understanding the foot."

IMAGING

MRI has been available as a diagnostic tool in veterinary medicine for more than 30 years and is the gold standard in evaluating problems of the equine musculoskeletal system. MRI units come in all sizes and shapes, allowing imaging of different parts of the equine body, resulting in higher-quality images. Basically, there are 2 major types: *closed-bore* MRI has a stronger and more stable magnetic field, resulting in better image quality; however, the size of the body region being imaged is the limiting factor in closed-bore systems. *Open-bore* MRI allows imaging of larger body regions with easier access and can be used in a horizontal or vertical configuration, allowing imaging in the sedated, standing horse. The vertical system is the preferred arrangement for imaging soft tissues of the distal extremity—especially the foot. There are low-gradient, field strength magnets 0.3 T or less (Tesla [T] being the unit of measurement for the different strengths of magnetic fields). High-grade, field strength magnets, better known as superconducting magnets, range from 1.5 to 3.0 T. These are the most common field strength magnets used in equine imaging. Dr Aitor Gallastegui will focus on the in-depth use of MRI and other imaging modalities for the equine foot.

Computed technology (CT) has also played an important role in advancing our understanding of the equine foot. *Cone beam computed tomography* (CBCT) uses divergent x-rays in a cone, in combination with CT, to create many images that can be anatomically reconstructed. This technology is used in equine orthopedics and sports medicine primarily for diagnostic purposes, and certain systems can image the foot in the standing horse. CBCT creates 400 to 600 images within minutes, producing a volume data set that software collects to reconstruct 3D images of the anatomic area. These anatomic data can be manipulated and visualized for surgery planning and treatment. Traditional CT (slice CT) or fan beam computed tomography (FBCT) has several similarities to CBCT, as well as important differences. For example, in FBCT the images are acquired slice-by-slice in 360° rotations as the patient moves perpendicular to the rotation, and the region of interest is imaged within seconds. Therefore, CBCT is more sensitive to motion artifact and has a decreased contrast resolution. CBCT has advanced to the point where imaging the foot is a reality. More details can be found in the article "*Imaging of the Foot.*"

Position emission is a more recent medical imaging technology that tracks the movement of radioactive-tagged compounds called radiotracers that have been injected into the body. Advanced scanners are being developed with a much higher sensitivity that can be used in clinical practice. The clinical applications are still evolving and should play an important game-changing role in diagnosing laminitis and other metabolic problems of the foot.

PAIN MANAGEMENT

Pain management relating to the equine foot has advanced over several decades because of a better understanding of the complex physiology and pathophysiology of pain; this has led to the classification of pain and applications to pain therapy. Pain classification in the horse uses a numeric system—types I, II, and III. Using this classification provides the clinician with better direction on how to approach pain therapeutically because the classification signifies the underlying biology and pathologic mechanisms in play. With this new information, primary care veterinarians and specialists in pain management have implemented a strategy called multimodal or balanced analgesia, compared with the past therapeutic approaches using the traditional, unimodal pain therapy. The multimodal or balanced analgesia entails using a combination of drugs with different mechanisms of action—often systemic, local, and regional approaches. The goal is to target the different sites of nerves conducting signals from the site of foot injury to the central nervous system and, hopefully, acting synergistically to attain the goal of analgesia and a restoration of homeostasis and function. Drs Driessen and Hopster will focus on managing foot pain in their article.

NUTRITION

After proper assessment of the patient's nutritional status at the time of injury, hospitalization, feeding the equine foot, and/or good dietary management of the entire patient affects morbidity, mortality, and the outcome of clinical cases. Take for instance the middle-aged to older horse developing insulin resistance in the case of endocrinopathic laminitis—better known as equine metabolic syndrome (EMS) and the many similarities to the same disease in people, human metabolic syndrome. Diet and exercise are 2 essential ingredients regulating and supporting normal insulin levels. Simple management practice, such as soaking hay, decreases nonstructural carbohydrate (NSC) levels, which helps reduce insulin levels and controls a disease like laminitis. Pasture grazing during certain times of the year—spring and fall with increased levels of NSC—puts horses with insulin resistance at risk for laminitis—emphasizing the importance of limiting grazing to earlier and later in the day, or simply using a grazing muzzle in this group of horses.

Initial assessment of nutritional status should include several steps. Body condition score (BCS) is a relatively simple and generally objective assessment of the nutritional status of the equine patient. Asking pertinent questions such as, "How is the horse's appetite?" tells a lot about the horse's general attitude and welfare, and, if affected, leads one to look further into whether there is some underlying physical, neurologic, or metabolic explanation for the change in appetite. Besides the horse with a poor BCS, using the Henneke body condition score of less than 3, ribs prominent, protruding vertebral processes, concave neck, and prominent sacrococcygeal area (tailhead), there is the overweight or obese horse with a BCS of 8 to 9 using the same scoring system. These equine patients develop hypertriglyceridemia and potentially life-threatening hyperlipemia—particularly in the pony, miniature horse, or donkey.

A dietary history is an important part of the nutrition evaluation, determining the types, amounts, and frequencies of feeds, forage, supplements, and pasture access. Forage evaluations that quantify NSC and other indicators of quality of the forage all help in assessing and determining a plan going forward. Like in other species, overweight or obese horses, as well as grossly underweight horses, place themselves in jeopardy for other systemic problems with potential effects on the immune system and organ functions. Dr Teresa Burns provides an in-depth overview on feeding the foot to maintain best health. If the foot is healthy, the odds are in favor that the rest of the horse will be as well.

CRYOTHERAPY

Few other anti-inflammatory therapies studied to date are as effective as simply cooling the foot. In the past 10 to 20 years, there have been several important developments in the use of hypothermia for the prevention and treatment of laminitis. It is well known that the mechanisms by which hypothermia protects the digital lamellae from injury during the developmental stage of laminitis are the result of a systemic inflammatory response. By blocking multiple inflammatory signaling pathways—central, upstream inflammatory signaling pathways—the many mediators of inflammation (chemokines and cytokines) are prevented from providing acute inflammation and subsequent degradation of lamellae tissue. Many newer practical methods have been developed for cooling the foot to achieve the evidence-based target temperature of 5°C and sustain the lamellar temperature less than 10°C for the duration of the laminitis risk period. It is well known that ice-water immersion boots, along with several dry-sleeve or boot systems, are successful in maintaining the lamellar temperature at or less than 10°C. Dr Daniella Luethy will update us on the principles of cryotherapy and the best systems currently available to successfully cool the foot and prevent and treat laminitis.

FOOT MECHANICS

The mechanics of the foot are as important, if not more so, than all the medical and surgical treatments that have been proposed to date. Rehabilitating the diseased foot or routinely managing the feet involves a combination of good physical evaluation along with needed radiographic examinations to direct the farrier in the appropriate trimming and shoeing. The physical examination of the foot entails hoof growth patterns, horn quality, and changes over time, changes in the coronary band that indicate load and stress on the lamellae tissue, and alignment of the hoof capsule and distal phalanx. The methodology and techniques are not as important as following appropriate principles. Radiographic assessment should include at least 2 orthogonal views. A lateral and dorsopalmar/dorsoplantar view depicts the position of the distal phalanx within the hoof and guides trimming and shoeing by the farrier. Foot mechanics will be an in-depth coverage from assessment to prophylactic techniques to maintain the foot in health and disease.

SUMMARY

The following are a list of references that will bring you up to speed on the many fabulous topics covered. I know each contributing author will share with you their expertise and specific references that apply to the points that are emphasized. Happy reading and continued good health to the equine foot.

DISCLOSURE

The author has nothing to disclose.

SUGGESTED READINGS

Alvarez AV, Schumacher J, DeGraves FJ. Effect of the addition of epinephrine to a lidocaine solution on the efficacy and duration of palmar digital nerve blocks in horses with naturally occurring forefoot lameness. Am J Vet Res 2018;79(10): 1028–34.

Amitrano FN, Gutierrez-Nibeyro SD, Schaeffer DJ. Effect of hoof boots and toe-extension shoes on the forelimb kinetics of horses during walking. Am J Vet Res 2016;77(5):527–33.

Angelone M, Conti V, Biacca C, et al. The contribution of adipose tissue-derived mesenchymal stem cells and platelet-rich plasma to the treatment of chronic equine laminitis: a proof of concept. Int J Mol Sci 2017;18(10):2122.

Armstrong C, Cassimeris L, Da Silva Santos C, et al. The expression of equine keratins K42 and K124 is restricted to the hoof epidermal lamellae of Equus caballus. PLoS One 2019;14(9):e0219234.

Bailey SR. Acute equine laminitis: exciting prospects afoot. Vet J 2015;206(2):121–2.

Bamford NJ. Clinical insights: treatment of laminitis. Equine Vet J 2019;51(2):145–6.

Barfoot C. Research sheds new light on laminitis risk factors. Vet Nurse 2016; 7(7):432.

Barstow A, Persson-Sjodin E. Science in brief: highlights from the equine abstracts at the Eighth International Conference on Canine and Equine Locomotion. Equine Vet J 2016;48(6):673–5.

Baxter GM. Supporting limb laminitis. Equine Laminitis; 2017. p. 210–3. Available at: https://onlinelibrary.wiley.com/doi/abs/10.1002/9781119169239.ch25.

Belknap JK. Laminitis: an overview. Equine Laminitis; 2017. p. 11–2. Available at: https://onlinelibrary.wiley.com/doi/abs/10.1002/9781119169239.ch2.

Belknap JK, Durham AE. Overview of laminitis prevention. Equine Laminitis; 2017. p. 421–6. Available at: https://onlinelibrary.wiley.com/doi/abs/10.1002/9781119169239.ch47.

Black B, Cribb NC, Nykamp SG, et al. The effects of perineural and intrasynovial anesthesia of the equine foot on subsequent magnetic resonance images. Equine Vet J 2013;3(45):320–5.

Bowker RM, Lancaster LS, Isbell DA. Morphological evaluation of Merkel cells and small lamellated sensory receptors in the equine foot. Am J Vet Res 2017; 12(29):659–67.

Buchner HHF, Peham C, Perrier J, et al. Effects of whole-body vibration on the horse: actual vibration, muscle activity, and warm-up effect. J Equine Vet Sci 2017; 51(51):54–60.

Byrne CA, Marshall JF, Voute LC. Clinical magnetic resonance image quality of the equine foot is significantly influenced by acquisition system. Equine Vet J 2020; 53(3):469–80.

Claerhoudt S, Bergman EHJ, Saunders JH. Computed tomographic anatomy of the equine foot. Anat Histol Embryol 2014;5(43):395–402.

Coleman MC, Belknap JK, Eades SC, et al. Case-control study of risk factors for pasture-and endocrinopathy-associated laminitis in North American horses. J Am Vet Med Assoc 2018;253(4):470–8.

Daniel AJ, Goodrich LR, Barrett MF, et al. An optimised injection technique for the navicular bursa that avoids the deep digital flexor tendon. Equine Vet J 2016; 48(2):159–64.

de Laat, Melody A, Reiche DB, et al. Incidence and risk factors for recurrence of endocrinopathic laminitis in horses. J Vet Intern Med 2019;33(3):1473–82.

Van Eps AW, Orsini JA. A comparison of seven methods for continuous therapeutic cooling of the equine digit. Equine Vet J 2016;48(1):120–4.

Van Eps AW, Pollitt CC. Digital hypothermia. Equine Laminitis; 2017. p. 306–15. Available at: https://onlinelibrary.wiley.com/doi/abs/10.1002/9781119169239.ch34.

Foreman JH, Bergstrom BE, Golden KL, et al. Dose titration of the clinical efficacy of intravenous flunixin meglumine in a reversible model of equine foot lameness. In: Proceedings of the 58th ann. Convention of the AAEP. 2012. p. 531–2.

Foreman JH, Foreman CR, Bergstrom BE. Acetaminophen/paracetamol efficacy in a reversible model of equine foot pain. Proceedings of the 62nd ann. convention of the AAEP. 2016. 295–6.

Gramberg K, Sunder A, Liebert F. Does the amino acid composition of the equine hoof horn correspond with the observed horn quality in horses?. In: Proceedings of the society of nutrition physiology. Gottingen, Germany: George-August-Universitat; 2017. p. 82.

Grundmann INM, Drost WT, Zekas LJ, et al. Quantitative assessment of the equine hoof using digital radiography and magnetic resonance imaging. Equine Vet J 2015;47(5):542–7.

Guedes A, Galuppo L, Hood D, et al. Soluble epoxide hydrolase activity and pharmacologic inhibition in horses with chronic severe laminitis. Equine Vet J 2017;49(3): 345–51.

Gutierrez-Nibeyro SD, McCoy AM, Selberg KT. Recent advances in conservative and surgical treatment options of common equine foot problems. Vet J 2018; 237:9–15.

Jordan VJ, Ireland JL, Rendle DI. Does oral prednisolone treatment increase the incidence of acute laminitis? Equine Vet J 2017;49(1):19–25.

Markwell HJ, Baxter GM. Prevention of supporting limb laminitis. Equine Laminitis 2017;427–31.

Mason JB, Gurda BL, Van Wettere A, et al. Delivery and evaluation of recombinant adeno-associated viral vectors in the equine distal extremity for the treatment of laminitis. Equine Vet J 2017;49(1):79–86.

Medina-Torres CE, Underwood C, Pollitt CC, et al. The effect of weightbearing and limb load cycling on equine lamellar perfusion and energy metabolism measured using tissue microdialysis. Equine Vet J 2016a;48(1):114–9.

Morgan J, Stefanovski D, Orsini JA. A novel dry ice crystal boot for cooling the equine digit. Vet Rec Open 2018;5:e000244.

O'Grady SE. Therapeutic shoes: application of principles. Equine Laminitis; 2017. p. 341–53.

Parks AH. Anatomy and function of the equine digit. Equine Laminitis; 2017. p. 13–21.

Shields GE, Barrett MF, Frisbie DD. Comparison of ultrasound and MRI for detection of soft tissue injuries in the palmar aspect of the equine foot. Proceedings of the 63rd annual convention of the AAEP, San Antonio, Texas. 2017. 208.

Trela JM, Spriet M, Padgett KA, et al. Scintigraphic comparison of intra-arterial injection and sital intravenous regional limb perfusion for administration of mesenchymal stem cells to the equine foot. Equine Vet J 2014;4(46):479–83.

Turner TA. Examination of the equine foot. Proceedings of the 64th annual convention of the American association of equine practitioners, san francisco, California, USA, 1-5 December 2018, Turner Equine Sports Medicine and Surgery, MN, USA, 340–346. 2018. Available at: https://aaep.org/sites/default/files/2018-12/Proceedings%2064th%20Annual%20Convention%202018_0.pdf.

van Eps, Andrew W, Burns TA. Are there shared mechanisms in the pathophysiology of different clinical forms of laminitis and what are the implications for prevention and treatment? Vet Clin North Am Equine Pract 2019;35(2):379–98.

Van Hamel SE, Bergman HJ, Puchalski SM, et al. Contrast-enhanced computed tomographic evaluation of the deep digital flexor tendon in the equine foot compared to macroscopic and histological findings in 23 limbs. Equine Vet J 2014;3(46):300–5.

Waguespack RW. Management of traumatic injuries to the equine foot. Proc North Am Vet Conf Large Anim 2010;289–91.

Wylie CE, Pollitt CC. In horses with chronic laminitis, do venograms compared to plain radiographs give greater diagnostic or prognostic information? Vet Evid 2017; 2(3):124.

Anatomy and Physiology of the Equine Foot

Mathew P. Gerard, BVSc, PhD

KEYWORDS

- Epidermis • Dermis • Hoof • Suspensory apparatus • Distal phalanx • Equine
- Anatomy

KEY POINTS

- The hoof integument is a structure of specialized epidermal, dermal, and subcutaneous tissues.
- An intact suspensory apparatus of the distal phalanx is critical to foot integrity and horse soundness.
- The neurovascular anatomy of the foot is a complex array of vessels and nerves, responding to regional and systemic inputs.

INTRODUCTION

Equus caballus has evolved from a small, multitoed, *Hyracotherium* ("Eohippus"), to the present-day single-toed and significantly larger ungulate.[1–3] Evidence of the multi-toed ancestors in today's horse may be more apparent than assumed.[4] The "foot" of ungulates is generally defined as the epidermal hoof capsule and all the tissues and structures enveloped by the capsule, including dermis, subcutaneous tissue, neuro-vascular tissues, bone, synovial spaces, tendon, ligament, and cartilage. The tremendous weight-bearing forces transmitted through the 4 digits of the horse are accommodated within physiologic norms because of the highly refined and specialized gross, microscopic, and functional anatomy of the equine foot. This article provides an overview of foot anatomy and physiology. There is overlapping, confusing, redundant, and highly varied terminology used for describing and identifying the foot structures of the horse.[5] Standardized anatomic language is derived from *Nomina Anatomica Veterinaria*[6] and the thoracic limb is used for directional and surface terms. When considering pelvic limb anatomy, "plantar" replaces "palmar."

BONES, CARTILAGE, LIGAMENTS

The third or distal phalanx (*phalanx distalis, os ungulare,* coffin or pedal bone), distal sesamoid bone (*os sesamoideum distale,* navicular bone) and distal part of the second

Veterinary Anatomy, Department of Molecular Biomedical Sciences, North Carolina State University, College of Veterinary Medicine, 1060 William Moore Drive, Raleigh, NC 27607, USA
E-mail address: mgerard@ncsu.edu

Vet Clin Equine 37 (2021) 529–548
https://doi.org/10.1016/j.cveq.2021.07.002
0749-0739/21/© 2021 Elsevier Inc. All rights reserved.

or middle phalanx (*phalanx media, os coronale*) are in the foot. The distal phalanx has 3 surfaces, 2 borders, and 3 processes (**Fig. 1**). The articular surface (*facies articularis*) principally contacts the articular surface of the head of the middle phalanx (*caput phalangis mediae*). Palmarly, a portion of the distal phalanx articular surface (*facies articularis sesamoidea*) is in contact with the distal sesamoid bone articular surface. The parietal (wall) surface (*facies parietalis*) is the dorsal surface of the distal phalanx, and this surface is suspended from the inner hoof wall. The extensive porosity of the parietal surface is indicative of the many neurovasculature structures passing between the bone and the overlying soft tissues.[7] The solear surface (*facies solearis*) of the distal phalanx is divided by the semilunar line (*linea semilunaris*) into a large and relatively flat area (*planum cutaneum*) that corresponds to the overlying sole region of the hoof and a smaller, roughened, flexor surface (*facies flexoria*) at the site of tendon and ligament insertions (see **Fig. 1C**). Adjacent to the flexor surface of the sole is the medial and lateral solear foramen (*foramen soleare mediale* and *laterale*), through which the digital arteries pass to enter the solear canal (*canalis solearis*) of the distal phalanx (see **Fig. 1C, D**). Shallow grooves in the bone (*sulcus solearis medialis* and *lateralis*) accommodate the digital arteries as they approach the solear foramina. The distal phalanx extends palmarly as the medial and lateral palmar processes (*processus palmaris medialis* and *lateralis*). On the proximal aspect of each process, a foramen (*foramen processus palmaris medialis* and *lateralis*) or a deep notch (*incisura processus palmaris medialis* and *lateralis*) with dorsal and lateral parts, is present (see **Fig. 1D**). Medial and lateral parietal grooves (*sulcus parietalis medialis* and *lateralis*) extend horizontally toward the dorsal midline of the distal phalanx from each respective process foramen or notch. Vessels travel in the grooves (see Hoof vasculature).

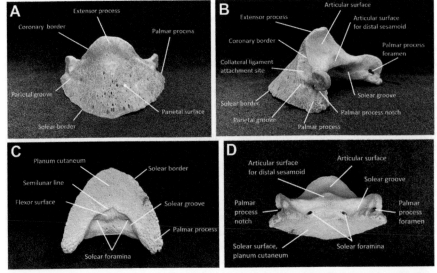

Fig. 1. (*A*) Dorsal view of a thoracic limb distal phalanx. Note the extensive porosity of the parietal surface. (*B*) Palmar oblique view of a thoracic limb distal phalanx. This specimen had a palmar process foramen on one side and a notch on the other side. (*C*) Solear surface of a thoracic limb distal phalanx. The solear surface is devoid of vascular foramina, except at the palmar processes. (*D*) Palmar and solear surface view of a thoracic limb distal phalanx.

The proximal border of the distal phalanx is the coronary border (*margo coronalis*) and at the dorsal midline this border rises to a peak at the extensor process (*processus extensoris*). The extensor process is the site of attachment of the common (long, in the pelvic limb) digital extensor tendon. At the distal edge of the distal phalanx is the solear border (*margo solearis*), and at its dorsal midline a shallow notch of the solear border (*crena marginis solearis*) is commonly found.[8]

The distal sesamoid bone has an articular surface with the distal and middle phalanges (**Fig. 2**). On the opposite, palmar side, is the flexor surface over which the deep digital flexor tendon (DDFT) passes, protected from the bone by the navicular bursa (*bursa podotrochlearis*). There is no anatomic term listed for the commonly described sagittal ridge of the flexor surface of the distal sesamoid bone. There is a proximal border (*margo proximalis*) and a distal border (*margo distalis*) to the distal sesamoid bone.

Extending from the medial and lateral palmar processes of the distal phalanx are the wing-shaped cartilages of the hoof (*cartilage ungularis medialis* and *lateralis*), commonly termed the "collateral cartilages." These cartilages have distal attachments along the semilunar line of the distal phalanx, fuse to the palmar surface of the DDFT, and project axially into the digital cushion over the bars of the hoof wall.[9] The ungual cartilages are mined by a network of vascular channels connecting venous plexuses.

Numerous ligaments support the foot. Medial and lateral collateral ligaments of the distal interphalangeal joint (*Ligg. collateralia*) extend from the distal phalanx to the middle phalanx. The distal sesamoid bone is connected to the proximal phalanx by the medial and lateral collateral sesamoidean ligaments (*Ligg. sesamoidea collateralia*), commonly referred to as the suspensory ligaments of the distal sesamoid bone (**Fig. 3B, C**). The distal sesamoidean impar ligament (*Lig. sesamoideum distale impar*, DSIL, distal navicular ligament) extends between the distal border of the distal sesamoid bone and the flexor surface of the distal phalanx, inserting immediately palmar to the DDFT (**Fig. 3A, C**). The insertion of the DDFT and DSIL is characterized by parallel, dense bundles of collagen, with septa of areolar tissue intervening. An abundant neurovascular network, including arteriovenous complexes, and elastic fibers are in the septal tissues, signifying important sensory and perfusion roles in the foot.[10,11] There are 5 ligaments attaching the ungual cartilages to bone or each other: cartilage to

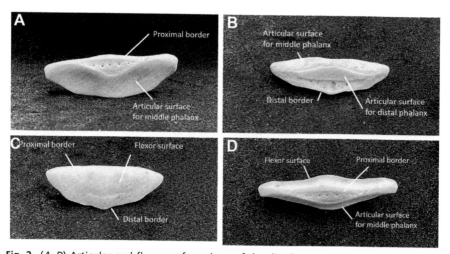

Fig. 2. (*A–D*) Articular and flexor surface views of the distal sesamoid bone.

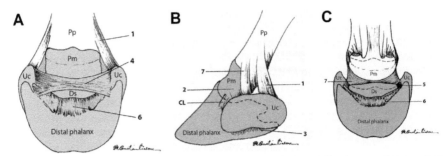

Fig. 3. (*A*) Palmar view of ligaments of ungual cartilages (Uc) and distal sesamoid bone (Ds). Pp, proximal phalanx; Pm, middle phalanx; 1, Ligg. chondrocompedalia; 4, Ligg. chondroungularia cruciate; 6, Lig. sesamoideum distale impar. (*B*) Lateral view of ligaments of ungual cartilages (Uc) and distal sesamoid bone. Pp, proximal phalanx; Pm, middle phalanx; CL, collateral ligament distal interphalangeal joint; 1, Ligg. chondrocompedalia; 2, Ligg. chondrocoronalia; 3, Ligg. chondroungularia collateralia; 7, Ligg. sesamoidea collateralia. (*C*) Deeper palmar view of ligaments of ungual cartilages (Uc) and distal sesamoid bone (Ds). Pm, middle phalanx; 5, Ligg. Chondrosesamoidea; 6, Lig. sesamoideum distale impar; 7, Ligg. sesamoidea collateralia. (*Adapted from* Constantinescu GM, Schaller O. Illustrated veterinary anatomical nomenclature, 3rd revised edition. Stuttgart: Enke Verlag. 2012. p 89; with permission.)

proximal phalanx (*Ligg. chondrocompedalia*), cartilage to middle phalanx (*Ligg. chondrocoronalia*), cartilage to palmar process of distal phalanx on same side (*Ligg. chondroungularia collateralia*), cartilage to palmar process of distal phalanx and cartilage of opposite side (*Ligg. chondroungularia cruciata*) and cartilage to distal sesamoid bone (*Ligg. chondrosesamoidea*) (see **Fig. 3**).

THE HOOF IN TOTO

The hoof (*ungula*), or "digital organ," includes epidermis, dermis, and subcutaneous tissues (hypodermis). The specialized hoof integument is continuous with the epidermis, dermis, and subcutaneous tissues proximal to the foot. The equine hoof is topographically subdivided into 5 or 6 segments: the limbic (ie, perioplic, in ungulates), coronary, parietal (wall), sole, and frog and heel bulb regions (**Fig. 4**). In artiodactyla (ruminants, pigs, deer, and antelopes), the frog and heel bulb regions are considered as 1 segment, the hoof pad. The periople (*limbus*) is the narrow zone of modified skin, between appendicular skin and the hoof, and this circumferential transition site is referred to as the coronet in ungulates. Immediately distal to, and continuous with the periople, is the coronary segment (*corona*), which is located proximally in the hoof and is the site of growth of the bulk of the hoof wall. The parietal segment of the hoof (*paries*) is distal to the coronary segment and includes the epidermal lamellae and the underlying dermis. Often, when referring to the "hoof wall" one implies the entire thickness of the cornified wall and is not specifically referring to the epidermal lamellae and associated dermis. The sole (*solea*), frog (*cuneus ungulae*), and heel bulb (*torus ungulae*) segments together occupy the ground surface of the foot and palmar region.

EPIDERMIS

Hoof epidermis is a well-organized mosaic of differently structured hard keratins (Gr *keras* horn), with regional variations in biomechanical properties and molecular

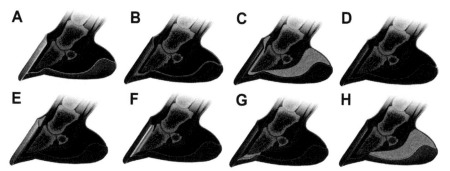

Fig. 4. (*A–H*) Integument of the foot by layer: epidermis (*A*), dermis (*B*), and subcutaneous tissue (*C*). Integument of the foot by region: limbic integument (*D*), coronary integument (*E*), parietal integument (*F*), solear integument (*G*), cuneate and bulbar integument (*H*). Image reproduced with permission from The Glass Horse: Elements of the Distal Limb; courtesy of ScienceIn3D.com. (*From* Parks AH. Anatomy and function of the equine digit. In: Belknap JK, Geor RJ, editors. Equine laminitis. Ames, Iowa: John Wiley & Sons, Inc; 2017. p. 13-21.; with permission.)

components. Production of the epidermis begins in its basal layer, the *stratum basale*. Cells of the basal layer migrate into the *stratum spinosum*. These 2 layers are called the germinal layer (*stratum germinativum*), or the "germinal epithelium," and this latter term is used when referring to the origins of epidermal tissue growth. As the epidermal cells migrate superficially, they undergo programmed modification to reach the keratinized state for their location.[12] The highly metabolically active germinal epithelium is nourished and sustained by the underlying dermis.

The epidermis of the hoof is the cornified hoof capsule (*capsula ungulae*). The hoof capsule wall (*paries corneus*) is divided into toe (*pars dorsalis*), lateral and medial quarters (*pars lateralis* and *pars medialis*), and lateral and medial heels (*pars mobilis lateralis* and *pars mobilis medialis*) regions. At the lateral and medial palmar angle of the wall (*angulus parietis palmaris lateralis* and *medialis*), there is an acute dorsal turn, and the wall continues from the heels as the bars (*pars inflexa lateralis* and *medialis*). The wall has a coronary border (*margo coronalis*) at its proximal edge, and a solear border (*margo solearis*) at its ground surface. In the heel region, a longitudinal ridge (*margo palmaris lateralis* and *medialis*) extends from the angle of the wall at the ground surface, to the coronary border. Two grooves are present internally, at the proximal extent of the cornified wall, and these grooves accommodate dermal tissues. The very narrow and shallow perioplic groove (*sulcus limbalis*) is immediately distal to the internal edge of the coronary border of the wall. The broader coronary groove (*sulcus coronalis*) lies distal to the perioplic groove.

The capsule wall consists of external, middle, and internal layers, that is, the *stratum externum*, the *stratum medium*, and the *stratum internum* (**Fig. 5**). The external layer (periople, or *epidermis perioplum [limbi]*) is formed by its germinal epithelium at the perioplic segment of the hoof. Proximally, the periople is a thickened, raised, approximately 1-cm-wide band of soft, unpigmented, tubular and intertubular horn (the colloquial "coronary band"). Distal to this band, the periople continues as a glossy, waterproofing film on the outer surface of the hoof wall, coating the wall as it grows toward the ground surface.

The middle layer forms the bulk of the capsule wall and is the primary load-bearing structure of the hoof at the ground surface. It is produced at the coronary segment of the hoof, by the germinal epithelium of the coronary epidermis (*epidermis coronae*).

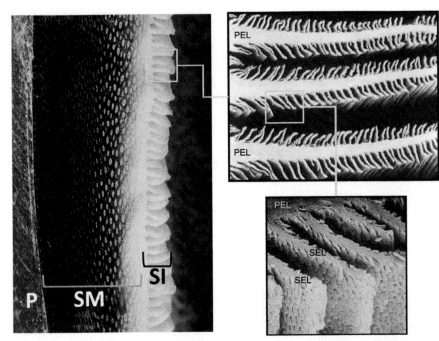

Fig. 5. Hoof wall layers. Stratum externum or periople (P) is the very thin outer wall layer. Stratum medium (SM, *light blue bracket*) forms the bulk of the hoof wall. The stratum internum (SI, *dark blue bracket*) is the epidermal lamellar layer consisting of primary epidermal lamellae (PEL) and secondary epidermal lamellae (SEL). Epidermal basal cells cover the surface of the SEL. (*Modified from* Pollitt CC. Anatomy and physiology of the inner hoof wall. Clin Tech Equine Pract 2004;3:4; with permission.)

The coronary epidermis is a lifelong cellular proliferating zone, producing keratinocytes that subsequently undergo maturation and ultimately cellular death, to form the middle horn of the wall.[13] The constant adding of keratinized epidermis at the coronary segment causes the middle layer to continuously move downward, past the distal phalanx to reach the ground surface. Average hoof growth is 6 to 8 mm/mo and is influenced by intrinsic and extrinsic factors. Whole body vibration increases hoof growth during its application, with no enduring effect following discontinuation of the modality.[14]

The middle layer consists of tubular and intertubular horn tissue. Hoof wall tubules are elongate, hollow cylinders of hard α-keratin, approximately 0.2 mm diameter.[15,16] Under circularly polarized light, tubule cortices exhibit 3 types of concentrically arranged layers of cells, and tubules vary in cross-sectional area and shape across the middle layer of the wall.[15] Tubules extend longitudinally and continuously in a parallel arrangement from their origin at the coronary segment to their contact with the ground surface. The tubular horn derives its cylindrical shape from the intimate association of its coronary germinal epithelium with the underlying template of coronary dermal papillae (*papillae dermales*). Visible, pin-point pocking of the slightly concave coronary groove identifies the conical holes that receive the dermal papillae scaffold (**Fig. 6**). The space between horn tubules is filled with intertubular horn derived from the germinal epithelium found between the pillars of dermal papillae. Intertubular horn may be pigmented or nonpigmented in the outer and middle regions of the middle

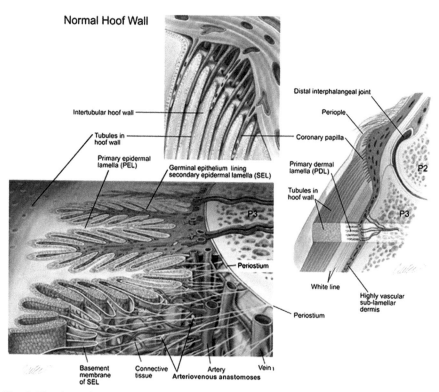

Fig. 6. The dermal papillae of the coronet and interdigitating lamellae of the inner hoof wall. (*From* Pollitt CC. The anatomy and physiology of the suspensory apparatus of the distal phalanx. Vet Clin North Am Equine Pract 2010;26(1):35; with permission.)

layer, but is consistently nonpigmented along a thin inner region, adjacent the internal layer of the hoof wall.[16] Horn pigmentation does not appear to affect mechanical behavior of hoof walls.[17,18]

The hoof wall keratin construct requires a certain degree of rigidity to avoid excessive deformation while accommodating, absorbing, and transferring the high loads of movement. On the other hand, the construct cannot to be too rigid, to avoid the risk of breaking. Mature keratinocytes are flattened, polygonal disks consisting of α-helical protein fibers (crystalline intermediate filaments [IFs]) embedded in a protein matrix.[12] Intramolecular and intermolecular disulphide crosslinks join the fibers and matrix together to form a stable composite. The alignment of IFs in keratin and the volume fraction of IFs affects the mechanical properties of the molecular structure.[19] A decreasing gradient of stiffness exists from the outer wall to the inner portion of the middle layer, allowing a controlled transfer of stress and strain loads from peak levels externally to the epidermal-dermal junction internally.[15,18,19] This stiffness gradient is a function of relative moisture content and changes in IF volume fraction in the keratin proteins.[15,19] Intertubular horn is oriented at large (sometimes right) angles to the axis of tubular horn. Variation in intertubular horn orientation and tubular horn morphology from outer to inner zones of the middle wall layer influences fracture toughness and fracture pathway propagation, providing a protective mechanism against wall cracks reaching sensitive deeper tissues.[15,17,20] In addition, variations in wall moisture content are associated with differing mechanical behaviors.[18,21,22]

Water gradients in the middle layer of the wall are supported by concurrent absorption of water through the tubular and intertubular horn.[23] The hollow tubules do not facilitate hoof hydration and likely contribute to dehydration through their exposed ends.[23,24] The middle layer is morphologically divided into 4 zones, based on tubule density measured at the center of the toe region (the "midline dead center") in the front feet of ponies and horses.[25,26] The most superficial zone (zone 1) has the greatest tubule density, and density declines in a stepwise manner, dorsopalmarly, to the innermost zone 4, adjacent the *stratum internum*. A mean tubule density of 15.6 tubules/mm^2 at the midline-middle of the wall was determined from transformed data for ponies and horses.[25,26] Tubule density has regional wall differences between the toe and quarter and between medial and lateral quarters.[27]

The nonpigmented, internal layer of the hoof wall, the *stratum internum*, features approximately 550 to 600 vertically arranged primary epidermal lamellae (PEL) (*lamellae epidermales*).[16] The lamellae extend in parallel rows from their proximal lamellar growth zone (at the inner shoulder of the coronary segment) to the ground surface of the wall.[7] Although mitosis of keratinocytes is primarily responsible for PEL growth, in newborn foals, bifurcation of lamellae is responsible for increasing PEL density at the toe region compared with the quarters.[28] The lamella shape represents a long thin rectangle, with the long edge extending from the coronary groove to the solear border. The short edge of the rectangle averages 3.58 mm in length, as measured in sectioned blocks created at a perpendicular plane (35° transverse plane) to the mid-dorsal hoof wall.[29] However, measured along the tensile axis of the suspensory apparatus of the distal phalanx (SADP) (at a 70° transverse plane), the lamellar length averaged 5.24 mm. This is the "true" lamellar length as it is measured along the same orientation of the functional axis of the SADP, and changes in this length may be considered a more accurate reflection of lamellar alteration.[29] Extending from each PEL are approximately 150 to 200 microscopic *secondary* epidermal lamellae (SEL) (**Fig. 7**). Secondary lamellae increase the anatomic surface area available for connection between the epidermal and dermal components of the hoof. This area averages 0.8 m^2, and the relative vastness of it helps to mitigate stress transfer from epidermis to bony column.[7] Although the PEL are completely keratinized structures, the SEL are not. SEL consist primarily of basal cells with ovoid nuclei lining a thin central, keratinized axis. The SEL have rounded club-shaped tips. The basal cells attach to a sheet of extracellular matrix, the basement membrane (BM), which intimately follows the contour of each SEL, demarcating this epidermal structure from the adjacent dermis (see Suspensory apparatus of the distal phalanx).[30,31] Secondary epidermal lamellae develop from proliferating basal cells at the proximal lamella growth zone.[13] The proliferating cells form folds along each PEL, and these folds elongate into secondary lamellae. Notably, epidermal lamellar keratinocytes do not undergo substantial cellular proliferation distal to their proximal growth zone origin. Rather, the continuous downward "flow" of the epidermal wall over the underlying dermis and distal phalanx relies on a complex molecular process of cellular reorganization.[32]

The cornified sole (*solea cornea*) segment of the hoof capsule develops from the germinal epithelium of the sole epidermis (*epidermis soleae*) and forms a large part of the capsule's solear surface (*facies solearis*). Like the hoof wall, tubular horn is embedded in intertubular horn in the sole. Horn tubules are modeled over dermal papillae projecting distally into the sole epidermis. As viewed from its normally concave external surface, the sole has a body (*corpus soleae*) located centrally and dorsal to the apex of the frog, and a medial and lateral "leg" (*crus soleae medialis* and *lateralis*), lying on either side of the frog. The sole has a wall border (*margo parietalis*) uniting with the internal side of the sole border of the hoof wall, and a central

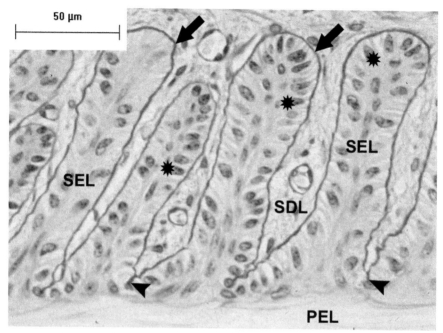

Fig. 7. Micrograph of normal hoof lamellae stained to highlight the BM. The BM (*arrowed*) of each SEL shows as a dark magenta line closely adherent to the SEL basal cells. Between the bases of each SEL the BM penetrates deeply (*arrowheads*) and is close to the anuclear, keratinized, PEL. The SEL tips are rounded (club-shaped). The basal cell nuclei are oval in shape (*stars*) and positioned away from the BM at the apex of each cell. The long axis of each basal cell nucleus is at right angles to the long axis of the SEL. The SDL are filled with connective tissue right to their tips, between the SEL bases. These parameters of hoof lamellar anatomy form the basis of the histologic grading system of laminitis histopathology. Stain: PAS. Bar = 10 μm. (*From* Pollitt CC. Anatomy and physiology of the inner hoof wall. Clin Tech Equine Pract 2004;3:16; with permission.)

border (*margo centralis*) with the frog. Unification of the sole and wall border epidermis occurs at the white zone (*zona alba*), discussed further in the Dermis section. The lateral and medial angles of the sole (*angulus soleae lateralis* and *medialis*) are the most palmar extremities of the sole legs, mirroring the adjacent angles of the hoof wall. Sole horn is thickest near the hoof wall and thinnest at the apex of the frog.

The final segment of the hoof epidermis is the pad of the hoof (*torus ungulae*), which is subdivided into 2 unique parts in the equine foot, the frog (*cuneus ungulae*) and heel bulbs (keeps the anatomic term *torus ungulae*). The frog and bulbar regions of the pad of the hoof are continuous with each other. The wedge-shaped frog segment in the horse is homologous to the apex of the pad of the hoof (*apex tori*) identified in swine and ruminants. The cornified frog (*cuneus corneus*) develops from the germinal epithelium of the epidermis of the frog (*epidermis cunei*). Again, tubular horn is embedded in intertubular horn in the frog. The frog has a dorsally directed apex (*apex cunei*), projecting into the sole, and a palmar base (*basis cunei*) located between the bars of the wall. Scarce merocrine glands discharge through the base of the frog. A medial and lateral crus of the frog (*crus cunei medialis* and *lateralis*) extends between the base and apex. The crura of the frog are deeply demarcated from the sole by grooves running along the side of the frog (*sulcus paracunealis lateralis* and *medialis*). On midline, the crura are separated by the central groove of the frog (*sulcus cunealis centralis*). The central groove is mirrored as a ridge on the internal surface of the frog, namely the spine of the frog (*spina cunei*) or the "frog stay." The frog stay projects proximally into the digital cushion of the foot. The cornified base of the frog continues palmarly as the rounded, medial, and lateral bulbs of the heel (*torus corneus, pars medialis* and *pars lateralis*), extending dorsal to the heels of the hoof wall, and completing the hoof capsule construct. The epidermis of the heel bulbs (*epidermis tori*) consists of relatively soft tubular and intertubular horn.

DERMIS

The dermis (or corium) is subdivided into segments matching the corresponding epidermis (**Fig. 8**). Perioplic dermis (*dermis limbi*) slots into the shallow perioplic groove of the proximal hoof wall. Perioplic dermal papillae, 1 to 2 mm long, project into the epidermis and provide a scaffold for tubular horn production. The perioplic dermis gradually widens toward the palmar aspect of the hoof and merges with the dermis of the heel bulb. The slightly convex band of coronary dermis (*dermis coronae*) nestles in the equally concave epidermal coronary groove. The coronary dermis, the overlying coronary germinal epithelium, and the underlying coronary subcutaneous tissue represent the anatomic "coronary band" of the foot. The coronary dermis is continuous proximally with the perioplic dermis and distally with the parietal dermis (*dermis parietis*). Laterally, the coronary dermis contacts the lateral surface of the ungual cartilages and palmarly it is continuous with the corium of the frog crura. Coronary dermal papillae, 4 to 6 mm in length, slot into individual holes in the epidermis. The surface of the papillae has parallel longitudinal ridges. It is inferred this feature increases the surface area of contact between the papillae and the germinal epithelium and may also provide channels to guide germinal keratinocytes into maturing proximo-distally oriented horn tubules.[7,30] The papillae taper to a blunt tip and decrease in density from the superficial to deep region of the coronary dermis, consistent with the varying zones of horn tubule density in the middle layer.[7,26] Coronary dermis transitions to parietal

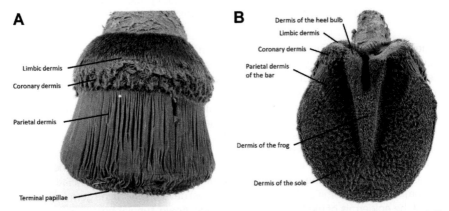

Fig. 8. (*A*) Dorsal view of dermis of preserved foot specimen. The limbic dermis is partially hidden by hair. The fine coronary papillae of the coronary dermis are clumped together in tufts. The parietal dermis consists of ~550 to 600 primary dermal lamellae, many adhered to each other in this wet specimen. (*B*) Solear view of dermis of preserved foot specimen. The dermis (corium) of the foot is continuous proximally with the appendicular dermis. The fine dermal papillae are clumped together in tufts. A portion of heel bulb is missing on the right.

dermis as this layer continues onto the parietal surface of the distal phalanx. Like the overlying epidermal lamellae, the parietal dermis is a construct of dermal lamellae (*lamellae dermales*) with primary and secondary components. Secondary dermal lamellae (SDL), compared with their epidermal counterparts, are narrow, with tapered tips that extend to within 1 to 2 epidermal basal cells of the axis of the PEL.[31] The dermal lamellae interdigitate with the epidermal lamellae forming the critical connection between the inner hoof wall and the dorsal surface of the distal phalanx.

It is important to reemphasize that although the parietal dermis is nourishing the overlying epidermal lamellae, continuous production of the stratum internum is occurring at the proximal lamellar growth zone (**Fig. 9**). After the cornified hoof wall passes the solear border of the distal phalanx and its attached dermal lamellae, there is no longer an interdigitation between the epidermal and dermal lamellae. At the distal edge of the dermal lamellae, a rim of 4 to 6-mm-long "terminal papillae" plug into the spaces previously occupied by the dermal lamellae (**Fig. 10**). Germinal epithelium at this location produces tubular and intertubular horn that seals the interlamellar gaps between the epidermal lamellae of this section of hoof wall, extending from the solear border of the distal phalanx to the ground surface. This seal is continuous with the adjacent solear epidermis, effectively forming the connection between sole and wall along the parietal border of the sole. At the ground surface, the tissue appears yellow due to the pigmentation of the horn produced at the level of the terminal papillae. This yellow section of epidermal lamellae and intervening horn between the solear border of the distal phalanx and the ground surface is known anatomically as the white zone or the white line of the hoof (*linea alba ungulae*). The innermost nonpigmented portion of the middle layer of the hoof wall may be included in the definition of white zone.[33] "White zone" was introduced as an anatomic term to avoid confusion with the "other" white line, that is, the ventral midline *linea alba* of the abdominal wall. "White line

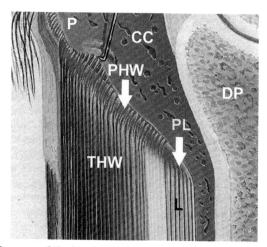

Fig. 9. The growth zones of the hoof (highlighted in *red*) are confined to the top or proximal region of the wall. Basal cells of the tubular hoof wall (middle layer of wall) and periople proliferate nonstop throughout the life of the horse. The proximal lamellae also proliferate at a rate similar to the hoof wall proper, but the rate is near zero in the lamellar regions below this. CC, coronary corium; DP, distal phalanx; L, lamellae; P, periople; PHW, proximal hoof wall; PL, proximal lamellae; THW, tubular hoof wall. (*From* Pollitt CC. Anatomy and physiology of the inner hoof wall. Clin Tech Equine Pract 2004;3:7; with permission.)

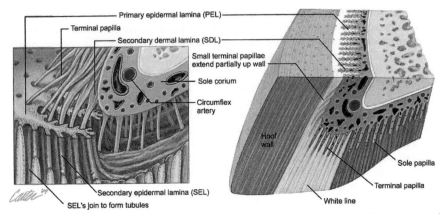

Fig. 10. On the distal end of all dermal lamellae are numerous terminal papillae. Germinal epidermis lining the terminal papillae are responsible for generating keratinized epidermal cells, which fill the space between the PEL as they grow toward the ground surface. (*From Pollitt CC. Anatomy and physiology of the inner hoof wall. Clin Tech Equine Pract 2004;3:11; with permission.*)

disease," as used in North America, is recognized as a misnomer, because it refers to pathology of the innermost nonpigmented part of the middle layer of the hoof wall, rather than of the white zone.[5,34]

Rounding the solear border of the distal phalanx, the parietal dermis continues onto the solear surface of the distal phalanx as the dermis of the sole (*dermis soleae*). The solear dermis adheres to the solear surface of the distal phalanx and has fine, short papillae that project into the epidermis of the sole. The solear dermis is continuous with the dermis of the frog (*dermis cunei*). The frog dermis is continuous with the dermis of the heel bulb region (*dermis tori*) (see **Fig. 8**B). As with the sole, the dermis of the frog and heel bulbs has fine papillae projecting into the overlying epidermis.

SUBCUTANEOUS TISSUES (HYPODERMIS)

Subcutaneous tissues are present in 3 of the hoof segments and form cushionlike structures in ungulates (see **Fig. 4**). In the horse, the perioplic subcutaneous tissue (*tela subcutanea limbi*), or perioplic cushion (*pulvinus limbi*), forms a narrow band deep to the perioplic dermis. The perioplic cushion is continuous distally with the coronary cushion (*pulvinus coronae*), that is, the subcutaneous tissue of the coronary segment (*tela subcutanea coronae*). The coronary cushion forms an outward bulging band of soft tissue, causing the coronary dermis to assume its convex contour. Subcutaneous tissue is not defined anatomically in the parietal segment, and a very thin subcutaneous tissue of the sole (*tela subcutanea soleae*) is inconsistently described. The modified hypodermis of the pad of the hoof (*tela subcutanea tori*) is better known as the digital cushion (*pulvinus digitalis*). In the horse, the digital cushion is divided regionally into a larger palmar part deep to the heel bulb dermis (*pars torica pulvini digitalis*) and a smaller frog part deep to the frog dermis (*pars cunealis pulvini digitalis*, or the *tela subcutanea cunei*). The digital cushion consists of variably distributed collagen bundles, elastic fibers, adipose tissue, vessels, nerves, and cartilage, with differences between breeds, and front feet versus hind feet.[9,35] Regional composition of the digital cushion has been correlated to the relative thickness of the ungual cartilages[9] and may also be associated with functional and adaptive differences of the digital cushion.[35] The digital cushion has a role in energy absorption and dissipation of applied forces and in the hemodynamic functions of the foot. Given a mechanical shock-absorbing role, one study described digital cushions as having surprisingly little adipose tissue and an abundance of interwoven collagen bundles in a myxoid tissue matrix rich in hyaluronan.[36]

SUSPENSORY APPARATUS OF THE DISTAL PHALANX

Apparatus suspensorius ossis ungulae includes all the structures establishing the suspension of the distal phalanx within the hoof of ungulates. The attachment anchors the parietal surface of the distal phalanx to the epidermal lamellae of the hoof capsule wall.[29,37] The connection is substantial; the SADP directs weight-bearing forces from the appendicular skeleton to the hoof wall and onward to the ground-bearing surface of the hoof wall, sparing the sole and frog/heel segments from primary force impact. At the epidermal attachment, the visible interweaving of the PEL and PDL shows the specialized junction between epidermis and dermis. The SEL and SDL projecting from each primary lamella markedly expand the surface area of contact between the interdigitating components. At the ultrastructure level, the key tissue connecting epidermis to dermis is the BM.[30–32,38] Akin to the pia mater intimately lining the central nervous system, the BM faithfully follows the contours of the lamellae, and epidermal and dermal structures attach to their respective side of the BM.

On the dermal side of the BM, bundles of collagen are arranged linearly along the longitudinal axis of the SADP. These collagen "cables" extend continuously from the distal phalanx, through the sublamellar dermis, into the PDL, and then finally the SDL, to reach the BM (**Fig. 11**).[29] The attachment of the collagen bundles to the distal phalanx is similar to a tendon to bone enthesis with 4 zones (fibrous connective tissue, uncalcified fibrocartilage, calcified fibrocartilage, bone) and a tidemark identified in the transition from soft tissue to bone.[39] The parietal surface of the distal phalanx has proximodistally oriented bone ridges, separated by intervening valleys. Rather than the collagen bundles attaching as a broad footplate across a relatively smooth bone interface, they are separated into an array of tiny tendrils that each attach to a point on a ridge of the distal phalanx, forming miniature tendonlike insertions.[29] Linear structures, consistent with Sharpey fibers, penetrate through the transition zones from distal phalanx ridgelines to osteoid matrix. Sharpey fibers are mechanically flexible due to the stretch and recoil properties of their component elastin. Their apparent presence and concentration along the bony crests support a suspensory construct with specific sites of high tensile stress. Given that Sharpey fibers are an extension of periosteum, it holds that the distal phalanx parietal surface is wrapped in (a somewhat fragmented) periosteum.[29]

At the dermal BM anchor point of the SADP, the collagen bundles become progressively smaller in size along the length of the PDL as fibers serially branch off to traverse SDL and reach their point of interweaving with the BM. The BM at the tip of the SEL has increased fiber insertion density, perhaps indicating this area experiences higher physiologic strain in the normal foot.[29] This observation may also explain the loss of BM attachment at the SEL tip as one of the early signs of lamellar pathology in laminitis.[29,31] The BM is a complex 3-dimensional mesh of collagen filaments (types IV and VII) and glycoproteins.[30,32] From the electron-dense layer of the BM, the lamina densa, numerous fibrils (some with hooklike configurations) extend into the matrix of the SDL and intermesh with type I collagen from the collagen bundles of the SADP. On the epidermal side of the BM, the electron-lucent layer, the lamina lucida, juxtaposes the plasmalemma of the epidermal basal cells of the SEL. Periodically,

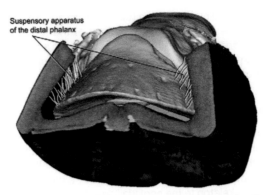

Suspensory apparatus
of the distal phalanx

Fig. 11. The distal phalanx is suspended within the hoof capsule by the suspensory appa-ratus. The SADP (a small part of which is shown here diagrammatically) attaches the entire parietal surface of the distal phalanx to the lamellae of the inner hoof wall. Diagram created from computed tomography data using MIMICS software (Materialise, Leuven, Belgium). (*From* Pollitt CC. The anatomy and physiology of the suspensory apparatus of the distal phalanx. Vet Clin North Am Equine Pract 2010;26(1):30; with permission.)

hemidesmosomes provide a bridging platform from the basal cell to the lamina densa. Extending from this molecular platform across to the lamina densa are fine microfila-ments (laminin glycoproteins). These microfilaments complete the attachment of the basal cells of the SEL to the BM, and hence on through the collagen fibers to the distal phalanx as described.

HOOF VASCULATURE

The arterial blood supply to the foot is in 3 zones with extensive communication be-tween the first (proximal dorsal) and second (distal dorsal) zones. The third, palmar or heel zone, does not anastomose with the dorsal zones.[40] Medial and lateral digital arteries (*Aa. digitales medialis* and *lateralis*) supply the foot with similarly named venous return vessels. Each digital artery, on its respective side, passes along the sol-ear groove and through the solear foramen of the distal phalanx, to enter the solear canal. The digital arteries anastomose within the solear canal, forming the terminal arch (*arcus terminalis*) (**Fig. 12**).

The digital pad branch (*ramus tori digitalis*) exits each digital artery at the level of the proximal interphalangeal joint. These vessels supply the palmar zone, including the dermis of the frog, heels, bars, and palmar perioplic and coronary regions, the digital cushion, ungual cartilages, DDFT, distal sesamoid bone, podotrochlear bursa, and distal interphalangeal joint.[7,16] The coronary artery (*A. coronalis*), arising from the dig-ital pad branch or the digital artery on each side, courses dorsally along the proximal border of the ungual cartilages and hoof capsule, and unites with its opposite. At the midlevel of the middle phalanx, the digital artery provides a dorsal branch of the mid-dle phalanx (*ramus dorsalis phalangis mediae*). This vessel courses dorsally on the axial side of the ungual cartilages and unites with its opposite. The coronary arteries and the middle phalanx dorsal branches distribute into the proximal dorsal zone, sup-plying the coronary and perioplic segments of the hoof, the proximal portion of the pa-rietal segment, the digital extensor tendon, and the distal interphalangeal joint. The palmar branch of the middle phalanx (*ramus palmaris phalangis mediae*) completes the arterial circle for the middle phalanx. At the level of the distal sesamoid bone, each digital artery supplies the dorsal branch of the distal phalanx (*ramus dorsalis*

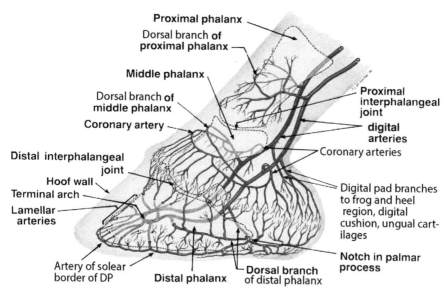

Fig. 12. The arteries of the equine foot. Design: C.C. Pollitt; Artwork: J. McDougall. (*Modified from* Pollitt CC. The anatomy and physiology of the suspensory apparatus of the distal phalanx. Vet Clin North Am Equine Pract 2010;26(1):38; with permission.)

phalangis distalis). These dorsal branches pass through the foramen or notch of the palmar process of the distal phalanx and then course dorsally within the parietal groove. These vessels supply the parietal segment of the quarters and heels and anastomose with the artery of the solear border of the distal phalanx (*A. marginis solearis*). The dorsal branch of the distal phalanx enters the parietal surface of the bone to anastomose with the terminal arch, and these 2 vessels are the principal blood supply for the distal dorsal zone.[16] From the solear canal, multiple small bony channels emanate like wheel spokes to distribute arterial branches from the terminal arch into and through the bone. Vessels perforating the parietal surface of the distal phalanx anastomose dorsally with vessels from the coronary segment. Distally, the branches feed into the artery of the solear border, and this vessel is the principal blood supply of the solear segment. The solear surface of the distal phalanx is devoid of vascular foramina, except at the palmar processes (see **Fig. 1**C). Therefore, the blood supply to the solear segment is dependent on the parietal vessels, wrapping over the solear border of the distal phalanx to join the solear border artery.

The microvasculature of the distal phalanx is regionally distributed with the greatest concentration of vessels at the solear border and a proportional decrease in osseous supply at the extensor process and midline region of the mid and proximal body of the distal phalanx.[41] This heterogeneous vessel concentration correlates with reported fracture healing in the distal phalanx. Solear border fractures have the best prognosis for healing, and fractures of the extensor process and midsagittal region of body of the distal phalanx have the poorest healing prognosis.

Venous return converges into the valved, medial and lateral digital veins (*V. digitalis medialis* and *lateralis*). Named larger veins of the hoof are satellite to the same named arteries. The coronary vein, the vein of the solear border, and the vein of the digital pad ("caudal hoof vein") receive anastomotic drainage from venous plexuses. A pair of veins parallels the arterial terminal arch within the solear canal, and these drain the deep venous network of the distal phalanx.[42] Valves in the intrinsic venous system of the foot are absent. In extrinsic veins, valves are confined to tributaries of the coronary veins and the digital pad veins and subsequently in the digital veins. The venous plexus of the hoof (*plexus ungularis*) is divided regionally into 3 extensive, interconnected venous networks.[7] The dorsal venous plexus is in the parietal segment, deep in the lamellar dermis. The coronary venous plexus occupies the coronary cushion of the coronary segment and extends over the abaxial surfaces of the ungual cartilages. The palmar venous plexus occupies the deep solear dermis and extends proximally along the axial surface of the ungual cartilage. The coronary and palmar plexuses anastomose through foramina in the ungual cartilages.[7,9]

The porosity of the parietal surface of the distal phalanx, beyond the 12 to 15 main foramina, is a consequence of the innumerable smaller foramina, through which vessels pass and form a meshwork within the overlying dermis. Gentamicin infused into the distal phalanx was detected in the extracellular fluid of the dermis, indicating the intimate relationship between the distal phalanx and parietal dermis vascular network.[43] Currently it is thought that disrupted perfusion to, and energy balance of, epidermal lamellar basal cells may be a contributor to the development of supporting-limb laminitis.[44] Cyclical limb loading, such as occurs during walking, promotes lamellar perfusion, whereas the effects of decreased limb loading frequency and increased weight bearing, as may occur in the natural state of supporting-limb laminitis, are less clear.[45] Axial arteries and veins traverse the dermal lamellae,[46–49] and these vessels are interconnected by arteriovenous anastomoses (AVAs) numbering approximately 500/cm² (**Fig. 13**).[49,50] The AVAs are larger and more concentrated at the base of the lamellae, have thick smooth muscle walls, and are innervated by an autonomic system network. The AVAs contribute to thermoregulation and pressure modulation in the hoof, allowing for rapid and effective shunting of blood to keep a digit warm or to bypass a high resistance capillary bed during peak loads on the foot (such as when galloping and jumping). AVAs are also located at the base of terminal and coronary papillae. All hoof dermal papillae, regardless of region, have a

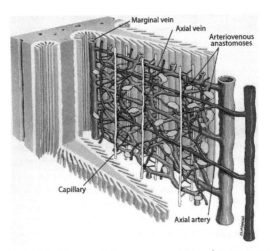

Fig. 13. The dermal microcirculation. AVAs are numerous and more concentrated near the bases of primary dermal lamellae. Secondary dermal lamella capillaries are shown reduced in number for diagrammatic reasons. (*Modified from* Pollitt CC. The anatomy and physiology of the suspensory apparatus of the distal phalanx. Vet Clin North Am Equine Pract 2010;26(1):42; with permission.)

similar structural organization consisting of a central artery and vein enmeshed in a cloak of capillaries.[47,49]

HOOF INNERVATION

Medial and lateral palmar (proper) digital nerves (*N. digitalis palmaris [proprius] medialis/lateralis*) innervate the parietal, solear, cuneate, and heel bulb segments of the hoof and the synovial, bone, cartilage, tendon, and ligament structures in the foot.[51–53] The dorsal branch(es) (*ramus dorsalis*) of the digital nerve exits at the level of the proximal sesamoid bones, tracks laterally and dorsally into the digit, and supplies the perioplic and coronary segments of the hoof.[52] The digital nerves pass into the solear canal, accompanying the vessels, and similarly distribute branches to the parietal surface of the distal phalanx. There is a rich network of sensory fibers and receptors in the foot, concerned with nociception, tactile and vibrational input, and vascular control.[10,11,50,54] Importantly, clinical experience shows that laminitic pain is not reliably blocked by a palmar digital nerve block alone, indicating the complexity of the sensory origins of the pain. In addition, the type of pain experienced, suggested to be neuropathic, may affect the response to perineural anesthesia. Pain arising from the coronary segment of the foot must be addressed by a dorsal branch block, and the more reliable reduction in laminitic pain following an abaxial sesamoid block substantiates the coronary segment as an important pain source in laminitis.

SUMMARY

The equine foot is a complex biological structure of functional significance to the integrity and well-being of the horse. A multitude of questions continue to drive research of this vital part of the horse anatomy. The following are just 2 examples where developing concepts require further scientific exploration and confirmation: how exactly are impact and load forces accommodated to avoid pathologic stress and fatigue of parts; and how exactly does epidermal hoof move past the stationary dermis and distal phalanx as it grows to the ground surface, while maintaining the dermoepidermal interface. As this *Veterinary Clinics* issue title implies, the needle is moving in the right direction.

DISCLOSURE

The author has nothing to disclose.

REFERENCES

1. MacFadden BJ. Fossil horses from "Eohippus" (hyracotherium) to equus: Scaling, Cope's law, and the evolution of body size. Paleobiology 1986;12(4): 355–69.
2. Floyd AE. Evolution of the equine digit and its relevance to the modern horse. In: Floyd AE, Mansmann RA, editors. Equine podiatry. St Louis (MO): Saunders Elsevier; 2007. p. 102–11.
3. McHorse BK, Biewener AA, Pierce SE. Mechanics of evolutionary digit reduction in fossil horses (equidae). Proc R Soc B 2017;284(1861):1174.
4. Solounias N, Danowitz M, Stachtiaris E, et al. The evolution and anatomy of the horse manus with an emphasis on digit reduction. R Soc Open Sci 2018;5(1): 171782.
5. O'Grady SE, Parks AW, Redden RF, et al. Podiatry terminology. Equine Vet Educ 2007;19(5):263–71.

6. International Committee on Veterinary Gross Anatomical Nomenclature. Nomina anatomica veterinaria. 6th edition. Editorial Committee, World Association of Veterinary Anatomists; 2017. Available at: http://www.wava-amav.org/. Accessed December 18, 2020.

7. Pollitt CC. Anatomy and physiology of the inner hoof wall. Clin Tech Equine Pract 2004;3(1):3–21.

8. Smallwood JE, Albright SM, Metcalf MR, et al. A xeroradiographic study of the developing equine foredigit and metacarpophalangeal region from birth to six months of age. Vet Radiol 1989;30(3):98–110.

9. Bowker RM, Van Wulfen KK, Springer SE, et al. Functional anatomy of the cartilage of the distal phalanx and digital cushion in the equine foot and a hemodynamic flow hypothesis of energy dissipation. Am J Vet Res 1998;59(8):961–8.

10. Van Wulfen KK, Bowker RM. Microanatomic characteristics of the insertion of the distal sesamoidean impar ligament and deep digital flexor tendon on the distal phalanx in healthy feet obtained from horses. Am J Vet Res 2002;63(2):215–21.

11. Van Wulfen KK, Bowker RM. Evaluation of tachykinins and their receptors to determine sensory innervation in the dorsal hoof wall and insertion of the distal sesamoidean impar ligament and deep digital flexor tendon on the distal phalanx in healthy feet of horses. Am J Vet Res 2002;63(2):222–8.

12. McKittrick J, Chen P-Y, Bodde SG, et al. The structure, functions, and mechanical properties of keratin. J Oncol Manag 2012;64(4):449–68.

13. Daradka M, Pollitt CC. Epidermal cell proliferation in the equine hoof wall. Equine Vet J 2004;36(3):236–41.

14. Halsberghe BT. Effect of two months whole body vibration on hoof growth rate in the horse: A pilot study. Res Vet Sci 2018;119:37–42.

15. Kasapi MA, Gosline JM. Design complexity and fracture control in the equine hoof wall. J Exp Biol 1997;200:1639–59.

16. Nickel R, Schummer A, Seiferle E. The circulatory system, the skin, and the cutaneous organs of the domestic mammals, vol. 3. Berlin and Hamburg, Germany: Springer-Verlag Berlin Heidelberg GmbH; 1981.

17. Bertram JE, Gosline JM. Fracture toughness design in horse hoof keratin. J Exp Biol 1986;125(1):29–47.

18. Douglas JE, Mittal C, Thomason JJ, et al. The modulus of elasticity of equine hoof wall: Implications for the mechanical function of the hoof. J Exp Biol 1996;199:1829–36.

19. Kasapi MA, Gosline JM. Micromechanics of the equine hoof wall: Optimizing crack control and material stiffness through modulation of the properties of keratin. J Exp Biol 1999;202:377–91.

20. Kasapi MA, Gosline JM. Strain-rate-dependent mechanical properties of the equine hoof wall. J Exp Biol 1996;199:1133–46.

21. Bertram JE, Gosline JM. Functional design of horse hoof keratin: The modulation of mechanical properties through hydration effects. J Exp Biol 1987;130:121–36.

22. Goodman AM, Haggis L. Regional variation in the flexural properties of the equine hoof wall. Comp Exerc Physiol 2009;5(3–4):161–8.

23. Sugimoto M, Kuwano A, Ikeda S, et al. Investigation of hydration processes of the equine hoof via nuclear magnetic resonance microscopy. Am J Vet Res 2012;73(11):1775–80.

24. Kasapi MA, Gosline JM. Exploring the possible functions of equine hoof wall tubules. Equine Vet J 1998;30(26):10–4.

25. Reilly JD, Cottrell DF, Martin RJ, et al. Tubule density in equine hoof horn. Biomimetics 1996;4(1):23–36.

26. Reilly JD, Collins SN, Cope BC, et al. Tubule density of the stratum medium of horse hoof. Equine Vet J 1998;30(26):4–9.
27. Lancaster LS, Bowker RM, Mauer WA. Equine hoof wall tubule density and morphology. J Vet Med Sci 2013;75(6):773–8.
28. Bidwell LA, Bowker RM. Evaluation of changes in architecture of the stratum internum of the hoof wall from fetal, newborn, and yearling horses. Am J Vet Res 2006;67(12):1947–55.
29. Pollitt CC, Collins SN. The suspensory apparatus of the distal phalanx in normal horses. Equine Vet J 2016;48(4):496–501.
30. Pollitt CC. The basement membrane at the equine hoof dermal epidermal junction. Equine Vet J 1994;26(5):399–407.
31. Pollitt CC. Basement membrane pathology: a feature of acute equine laminitis. Equine Vet J 1996;28(1):38–46.
32. Pollitt CC. The anatomy and physiology of the suspensory apparatus of the distal phalanx. Vet Clin North Am Equine Pract 2010;26(1):29–49.
33. Budras K-, Hullinger RL, Sack WO. Light and electron microscopy of keratinization in the laminar epidermis of the equine hoof with reference to laminitis. Am J Vet Res 1989;50(7):1150–60.
34. O'Grady SE, Burns TD. White line disease: a review (1998-2018). Equine Vet Educ 2021;33(2):102–12.
35. Faramarzi B, Lantz L, Lee D, et al. Histological and functional characterizations of the digital cushion in quarter horses. Can J Vet Res 2017;81(4):285–91.
36. Egerbacher M, Helmreich M, Probst A, et al. Digital cushions in horses comprise coarse connective tissue, myxoid tissue, and cartilage but only little unilocular fat tissue. Anat Histol Embryol 2005;34(2):112–6.
37. Budras K, Hirschberg R, Hinterhofer C, et al. The suspensory apparatus of the coffin bone - part 1: The fan-shaped re-inforcement of the suspensory apparatus at the tip of the coffin bone in the horse. Pferdeheilkunde 2009;25(2):96–104.
38. Pollitt CC, Daradka M. Equine laminitis basement membrane pathology: Loss of type IV collagen, type VII collagen and laminin immunostaining. Equine Vet J 1998;30(S26):139–44.
39. Apostolakos J, Durant TJ, Dwyer CR, et al. The enthesis: a review of the tendon-to-bone insertion. Muscles Ligaments Tendons J 2014;4(3):333–42.
40. Parks AH. Anatomy and function of the equine digit. In: Belknap JK, Geor RJ, editors. Equine laminitis. Ames (IA): John Wiley & Sons, Inc; 2017. p. 13–21.
41. Schade SM, Arnoczky SP, Bowker RM, et al. The microvasculature in the equine distal phalanx: implications for fracture healing. Vet Comp Orthop Traumatol 2014;27(2):102–6.
42. Mishra PC, Leach DH. Extrinsic and intrinsic veins of the equine hoof wall. J Anat 1983;136(Pt 3):543–60.
43. Nourian AR, Mills PC, Pollitt CC. Development of intraosseous infusion of the distal phalanx to access the foot lamellar circulation in the standing, conscious horse. Vet J 2010;183(3):273–7.
44. van Eps AW, Burns TA. Are there shared mechanisms in the pathophysiology of different clinical forms of laminitis and what are the implications for prevention and treatment? Vet Clin North Am Equine Pract 2019;35(2):379–98.
45. Medina-Torres CE, Underwood C, Pollitt CC, et al. The effect of weightbearing and limb load cycling on equine lamellar perfusion and energy metabolism measured using tissue microdialysis. Equine Vet J 2016;48(1):114–9.
46. Mishra PC, Leach DH. Electron microscopic study of the veins of the dermal lamellae of the equine hoof wall. Equine Vet J 1983;15(1):14–21.

47. Nasu T, Yamanaka T, Nakai M, et al. Scanning electron microscopic study of the vascular supply of the equine hoof. J Vet Med Sci 1998;60(7):855–8.
48. Hirschberg RM, Bragulla HH. Functional considerations regarding the angioarchitecture of the equine hoof. Pferdeheilkunde 2007;23(1):27–38.
49. Pollitt CC, Molyneux GS. A scanning electron microscopical study of the dermal microcirculation of the equine foot. Equine Vet J 1990;22(2):79–87.
50. Molyneux GS, Haller CJ, Mogg K, et al. The structure, innervation and location of arteriovenous anastomoses in the equine foot. Equine Vet J 1994;26(4):305–12.
51. Schumacher J, Schramme MC, Schumacher J, et al. Diagnostic analgesia of the equine digit. Equine Vet Educ 2013;25(8):408–21.
52. Paz CFR, Magalhães JF, Mendes HMF, et al. Mechanical nociceptive thresholds of dorsal laminae in horses after local anaesthesia of the palmar digital nerves or dorsal branches of the digital nerve. Vet J 2016;214:102–8.
53. Budras K, Sack WO, Rock S, et al. Anatomy of the horse. 6th edition. Hannover, Germany: Schlutersche Verlagsgesellschaft mbH & Co. KG.; 2011. p. 26–9.
54. Bowker RM, Lancaster LS, Isbell DA. Morphological evaluation of Merkel cells and small lamellated sensory receptors in the equine foot. Am J Vet Res 2017; 78(6):659–67.

Pharmacology of the Equine Foot

Medical Pain Management for Laminitis

Klaus Hopster, DVM, PhD, DiplECVAA*,
Bernd Driessen, DVM, PhD, Dipl ACVAA, Dipl ECVPT

KEYWORDS

- Analgesia • Dexmedetomidine • Epidural • Horse • Laminitis • Opioid

KEY POINTS

- Nonsteroidal anti-inflammatory drugs remain the foundation for the successful management of laminitis pain.
- Newer α-2 agonists such as dexmedetomidine might not only provide strong analgesia, but also have tissue-protective effects.
- Epidural analgesia not only involving caudal but also cervical epidural catheters offers a new possibility for strong analgesia with fewer drug-related side effects.

INTRODUCTION, HISTORY, DEFINITIONS, AND BACKGROUND

Laminitis is inflammation and injury of the tissue between the hoof and the underlying coffin bone that causes the interdigitating laminae of the hoof wall to separate. In severe cases, laminitis can progress to founder, in which the injured tissue loses the ability to suspend the body weight of the horse within the hoof capsule and therefore the hoof and coffin bone are separated. In these cases, the coffin bone generally rotates or sinks, leading to severe pain. Therefore, one of the most important components in the management of the laminitic patients is the control of pain and improved analgesic therapy.

SYSTEMIC MANAGEMENT
Nonsteroidal Anti-inflammatory Drugs

The foundation of most therapeutic protocols for laminitis treatment has been and continues to be the treatment with nonsteroidal anti-inflammatory drugs (**Table 1**).

Briefly, most NSAIDs act as nonselective inhibitors of the cyclo-oxygenase (COX) enzymes. This inhibition is competitively reversible, as opposed to the mechanism of aspirin, which causes irreversible inhibition.[1] The COX catalyze the formation of

Department of Clinical Studies, School of Veterinary Medicine, University of Pennsylvania, 382 West Street Road, Kennett Square, PA 19348, USA
* Corresponding author.
E-mail address: khopster@upenn.edu

Vet Clin Equine 37 (2021) 549–561
https://doi.org/10.1016/j.cveq.2021.08.004
0749-0739/21/© 2021 Elsevier Inc. All rights reserved.

vetequine.theclinics.com

Table 1
Dose recommendations for analgesic drugs systemically used for pain management in horses with laminitis

Drug	Dose
Flunixin–meglumine	1.1 mg/kg IV/PO q12–24h (BID–SID)
Phenylbutazone	2.2–4.4 mg/kg IV/PO q12–24h (BID–SID)
Ketoprofen	2.2–3.6 mg/kg IV/IM q6–24h (QID–SID)
Meloxicam	0.6 mg/kg IV/PO q24 h (SID)
Firocoxibe	0.1 mg/kg PO q24 h (SID)
Detomidine	0.005–0.03 mg/kg IV/IM every 3–4 h
Dexmedetomidine	1.5–3.0 μg/kg IV/IM every 3–4 h CRI at 0.75–1.8 μg/kg/h
Morphine	0.1–0.2 mg/kg IV/IM every 4–6 h
Methadone	0.1–0.2 mg/kg IV/IM q6h (QID)
Butorphanol	0.01–0. 4 mg/kg IV/IM every 2–3 h CRI 15–25 μg/kg/h
Gabapentin	5–20 mg/kg PO q8–12h (TID–BID)
Lidocaine	Bolus of 1.5 mg/kg over 10 min followed by 3 mg/kg/h
Ketamine	0.3–0.6 mg/kg/h IM/IV CRI

Routes and intervals of drug administration: IV, intravenous; IM, intramuscular; PO, per os; SID, once daily; BID, twice daily; TID, three times daily; QID, four times daily.

prostaglandins and thromboxane from arachidonic acid, which act as messenger molecules in the inflammatory process.

However, many aspects of the analgesic mechanism of NSAIDs remain unexplained and, for this reason, additional COX pathways are hypothesized to be involved. The COX-3 pathway was believed to explain this discrepancy; however, recent studies make it seem unlikely that it plays any major role in humans and alternative explanation models are proposed.[2]

NSAIDs interact with the endocannabinoid system and its endocannabinoids. COX-2 has been shown to use endocannabinoids as substrates and may play a key role in both the therapeutic and adverse effects of NSAIDs, as well as NSAID-induced placebo responses.[3–5]

Evidence of increased COX expression, leukocyte migration, and cytokine production in the developmental and acute phases of laminitis indicate that NSAID therapy is most beneficial before the onset of lameness during the early (developmental) stages of the disease. However, there is increasing evidence to suggest that commonly administered NSAIDs such as phenylbutazone and flunixin meglumine do not only mediate their effects through anti-inflammatory action in the affected tissues, but also produce analgesia by the inhibition of central sensory neurons through COX-dependent and other independent mechanisms.[6–9]

Although NSAID administration in higher doses to achieve anti-inflammatory activity is desirable in the early stage of laminitis, the pain relief from NSAIDs must be balanced against the risks of exacerbated structural injury owing to excessive movement and limb loading.[6,10] To avoid causing further injury, the dose should be titrated based on the comfort level of the patient. In horses with chronic laminitis, effective analgesia frequently calls for high doses of NSAIDs and an effect may still not be seen for up to 3 days after the start of treatment.[6] This point must be considered when assessing the clinical response to NSAIDs.

The previously held belief that more COX-2–preferential or even –selective NSAIDS are therapeutically superior has been recently challenged.[11–13] New data indicate that the suppression of inflammation-evoked central nociceptive activity and hyperalgesia by NSAIDs may be related to the selectivity for COX isoforms. COX-2 seems only to be involved in the initiation, but not necessarily the maintenance, of nociceptive spinal neuron activation, which may largely depend on COX-1.[14] Assuming that inflammation is the common pathologic denominator in all forms of laminitis and therefore the trigger for increased spinal sensory nerve excitability, these laboratory findings suggest that nonselective NSAIDs are more effective for analgesic therapy in laminitis.

Owing to the complexity of laminitis pain and the potential side effects, multimodal combinations based on NSAIDs combined with other analgesics (as discussed elsewhere in this article) are recommended to achieve a decrease in NSAID dose requirements in individual cases at different stages of the disease, decreasing the risk of NSAID-related side effects.

Opioids

Opioids are among the oldest drugs used to relieve pain. However, it is only recently that the mechanisms underlying their analgesic actions have been better understood. In the past 2 decades, huge advancements have been made in this field.

Opioid drugs mimic the actions of the endogenous opioid peptides by interacting with specific receptors, the opioid receptors, to produce a variety of pharmacologic effects. Currently, 3 distinct opioid receptor types, μ (mu), δ (delta), and κ (kappa), are recognized and all have recently been cloned.[15] The μ receptor is important in sensory processing, including the modulation of nociceptive stimuli, extrapyramidal functioning, and limbic and neuroendocrine regulation. There are 2 subtypes of the μ receptor, a high-affinity μ receptor and a low-affinity $\mu2$ receptor.[15] Two subtypes of the δ receptor and 3 subtypes of the κ receptor have also been described.[15] The supraspinal mechanisms of analgesia produced by μ opioid agonist drugs is thought to involve the $\mu1$ receptor, whereas spinal analgesia, respiratory depression, and the gastrointestinal effects of opioids are associated with the $\mu2$ receptor.

The opioid receptors are G-protein–coupled receptors that influence different second messenger pathways.[16] The actions of opioids are primarily inhibitory by closing voltage-operated calcium channels and opening calcium-dependent potassium channels. This process results in the hyperpolarization and decrease in neuronal activity and excitability.[17] Opioids can also have excitatory effects involving both the disinhibition of interneurons and direct excitation of neurons themselves. Nanomolar concentrations, acting via G proteins, stimulate adenylyl cyclase activity in certain neurons.[18] This process may be responsible for some responses to opioids, such as excitement, aggression, paradoxic hyperalgesia, and pruritus.

Opioids selectively modulate the pain sensation carried by slowly conducting, unmyelinated C fibers, but have little effect on sharp pain carried by small, myelinated Aδ fibers. In the dorsal horn, transmission of peripheral nociceptive signals via C fiber neurons involves the presynaptic release of neuropeptides such as substance P, neurokinin A, and glutamate. These neuropeptides bind to postsynaptic receptors, such as AMPA and N-methyl-D-aspartate (NMDA) receptors, leading to depolarization and changes in second messengers.[19] Opioids also directly hyperpolarize the postsynaptic membranes of dorsal horn neurons. They also interfere with the action of prostaglandins at peripheral sites, and μ agonists particularly inhibit prostaglandin E2–induced hyperalgesia in a dose-dependent fashion.[20]

The use, particularly the long-term use, of opioids in horses has been controversial owing to the decrease in gastrointestinal motility commonly seen as a side effect, which may predispose horses to the development of abdominal pain (colic). The incorporation of opioid therapy into the regular management of laminitis is likely to require the development and validation of novel agents in the horse.

α-2 Agonists

The primary mechanism of action of α-2 agonists is stimulation of presynaptic α-2 adrenoceptors in the central nervous system, activating inhibitory neurons that lead to a decrease in sympathetic output via a negative feedback mechanism.[21]

Through a second messenger cascade, the stimulation of α-2 adrenoceptors, coupled with G-protein, leads to an inhibition of adenylate cyclase and subsequently to an intracellular decrease in cyclic adenosine monophosphate. Activation of α-2 adrenoceptors leads to opening of potassium channels and the subsequent outflow of potassium. This process causes hyperpolarization and makes the cell insensitive to excitatory stimuli in the central and peripheral nervous systems.[22] Further, it can suppress the calcium influx at the voltage-dependent calcium channel of the terminal nerve endings. The latter mechanism is responsible for the presynaptic inhibition of the release of neurotransmitters such as noradrenaline (negative feedback).[23] The α-2 adrenoceptors are found in both the central nervous system and peripheral tissues, which explains the central analgesic effects as well as the peripherally mediated side effects.[24]

Dexmedetomidine is a highly selective α-2 agonist. There is increasing evidence suggesting that dexmedetomidine has further organ-protective effects, including of the kidney, brain, and heart[25] A recently published study was able to demonstrate that dexmedetomidine given to horses either before or after the occurrence of an ischemic event significantly decreased small intestine injury.[26,27] Although the protective mechanism of dexmedetomidine against ischemia–reperfusion injury remains unclear, it has been speculated that dexmedetomidine could have protective effects on the lamellae in laminitic horses by decreasing the degree of ischemia induced necrosis.

Gabapentin

Gabapentin was designed to mimic the neurotransmitter GABA. It does, however, not bind to GABA receptors. Its mechanism of action as an antiepileptic agent involves the inhibition of the α-2-delta subunit of voltage-gated calcium channels.[28] In human medicine, gabapentin is recommended as a treatment for chronic neuropathic pain.[29,30]

In horses, gabapentin has a relatively low oral bioavailability of approximately 16% with an elimination half-life of about 8.5 hours.[31] This property equals high dosages and frequent application intervals are needed to maintain sufficient and constant plasma levels. Horses tolerated dosages of up to 20 mg/kg gabapentin well and showed only mild signs of sedation.[31]

Published reports indicate good efficacy of gabapentin when used as an adjunctive analgesic for the treatment of neuropathic pain such as laminitis.[32] In contrast, in a recently published study, gabapentin did not improve subjective or objective measures of lameness when administered to horses with chronic thoracic limb lameness.[33] The authors discussed that even higher oral doses than the 20 mg/kg and longer treatment regimens of gabapentin may be necessary for the effective treatment of chronic musculoskeletal pain in horses.

Ketamine

Ketamine is a phencyclidine derivative that was developed in the 1960s as an anesthetic agent. The most important pharmacologic properties of ketamine are its function as a noncompetitive N-methyl-D-aspartate receptor antagonist, and its analgesic action at subanesthetic dose is believed to be primarily owing to the N-methyl-D-aspartate receptor antagonism in the brain and spinal cord.[34] Ketamine also interacts with other receptors and channels, including nicotinic and muscarinic acetylcholine receptors, opioid receptors, monoaminergic receptors, and voltage-sensitive sodium channels.[35]

Further, ketamine has anti-inflammatory effects, modulating the production of different proinflammatory mediators. A recent study using a rabbit model of gonarthrosis (arthritis of the knee) found that ketamine suppressed the inflammatory response in osteoarthritis,[36] whereas a systematic review concluded that intraoperative ketamine reduces the postoperative IL-6 inflammatory response in surgical patients.[37]

Ketamine has been used in horses to treat chronic and acute pain. Dosages of up to 0.5 mg/kg as a bolus or 1 mg/kg/h as a continuous infusion have shown to have antinociceptive effects in horses without causing significant side effects or ataxia.[38,39] Although the analgesic effects of ketamine as a sole agent are limited, it has been shown to induce analgesia when used in subanesthetic doses in horses with chronic laminitis.[40] For this reason, ketamine can be combined with other drugs such as α-2 agonists and/or opioids as part of a multimodal analgesic approach.

Lidocaine

The systemic administration of the local anesthetic lidocaine has been shown to be antinociceptive in both acute and chronic pain states, especially in acute postoperative and chronic neuropathic pain. These effects cannot be explained by its voltage-gated sodium channel blocking properties alone. The responsible mechanisms remain elusive with multiple theories proffered in the literature.

Several in vitro studies confirmed that lidocaine inhibits GABA release and GABA-induced chloride currents.[41,42] In contrast, in vitro lidocaine potentiates GABA-mediated chloride currents by inhibiting GABA uptake.[43] This factor may explain the antinociceptive effects of lidocaine, given that other GABA uptake inhibitors, such as tiagabine, have well-documented beneficial effects in chronic pain.[44]

Neuroinflammation is associated with the induction and maintenance of chronic pain with non-neuronal cells playing a key role.[45] The activation and infiltration of leucocyte-activated glial cells and the production of inflammatory mediators both drive inflammatory signaling cascades that lead to the activation of nociceptors. Lidocaine affects inflammatory cells in vitro in many ways,[46,47] including the inhibition of priming of human peripheral polymorphonuclear cells or neutrophils.[48,49] Lidocaine can furthermore reduce the release of mediators of inflammation, such as IL-4, IL-6, and tumor necrosis factor-α.[50–54]

Another explanation of the analgesic properties of systemic lidocaine is that lidocaine inhibits dose-dependent nitric oxide production.[55] Furthermore, it inhibits inducible nitric oxide synthase, possibly by a mechanism involving voltage-gated sodium channels.[56] More recently, suppression of L-arginine uptake was shown to underlie the inhibitory effects of lidocaine on nitric oxide synthesis.[57] Lidocaine also inhibits the tumor necrosis factor-α–induced activation of endothelial nitric oxide synthase in lung microvascular endothelial cells, which prevents nitric oxide production and further propagation of inflammatory signaling.[58]

Amitriptyline

Amitriptyline is a tricyclic antidepressant. The efficacy of tricyclic antidepressants to relieve neuropathic pain first emerged from observations in depressed patients treated with imipramine.[59] Since the 1980s, clinical trials have confirmed the benefit of amitriptyline to relieve postherpetic neuropathic pain and painful diabetic polyneuropathy.[60] This effect occurs independently from the presence of a depressive syndrome.[61] Moreover, the relief of neuropathic pain may also be observed without modification of the depression scores,[62] and at lower doses than necessary to treat major depression. Unlike classical analgesics, the effect of antidepressants on neuropathic pain is observed after prolonged treatment, suggesting the involvement of neuronal plasticity; however, no evidence of a dose–response effect could be shown. In human medicine, the described side effects from therapy with amitriptyline are drowsiness, dizziness, dry mouth, constipation, nausea, urinary retention, sweating, headache, blurred vision, palpitations, irritability, and ataxia. There are currently no studies in horses demonstrating the efficacy of amitriptyline in laminitis.

Soluble Epoxide Hydrolase Inhibitor

Among the novel anti-inflammatory and analgesic medications under investigation, a soluble epoxide hydrolase inhibitor has shown some promising results. Cytochrome P450 epoxygenases mediate a relatively unexplored pathway of arachidonic acid by which endogenous bioactive lipids, known as epoxy fatty acids, are produced.[63] A downstream enzyme, soluble epoxide hydrolase, metabolizes the epoxy fatty acids into the corresponding diols.[64] The diols are less active or inactive in terms of antinociception.[65] It has been shown that pharmacologic inhibition of soluble epoxide hydrolase results in stabilization of epoxy fatty acids and antinociceptive effects more significantly than after treatment with COX inhibitors, opioids, or gabapentin.[65] In the spinal cord, soluble epoxide hydrolase inhibition results in epoxy fatty acid–mediated downregulation of COX-2 transcription and rapid upregulation of the acute neurosteroid-producing gene in the presence of elevated cyclic adenosine monophosphate levels, which then results in neurosteroid production and analgesia via GABA channels.[66] The arachidonic acid–derived epoxy fatty acids also produce analgesia via activation of β-endorphin and met-enkephalin in the ventrolateral periaqueductal gray matter.[67] In peripheral neurons, soluble epoxide hydrolase inhibitors decrease endoplasmic reticulum stress, resulting in the amelioration of neuropathic pain more efficiently than gabapentin.[68]

A recent study reported that soluble epoxide hydrolase activity was significantly increased in horses with active chronic laminitis compared with healthy horses. Additionally, it was shown that several inhibitors designed to inhibit the human enzyme are also active against equine soluble epoxide hydrolase.[69] Adjunct therapy with 4-(4-(3-(4-trifluoromethoxy-phenyl)ureido)cyclohexyloxy)benzoic acid (t-TUCB), a potent pharmacologic epoxide hydrolase inhibitor, in horses with severe chronic laminitis resulted in mild to moderate, statistically significant decreases in thoracic limb lifts and pain scores, suggesting that t-TUCB helped to control the pathologic pain associated with laminitis.[70] These results reason for a role of endogenous bioactive lipids in laminitis pain signaling and support the further exploration into manipulating these molecules, via soluble epoxide hydrolase inhibition or other strategies, as an additional therapeutic approach for laminitis.

LOCAL THERAPEUTIC OPTIONS
Caudal Epidural Catheter

Epidural analgesia is the administration of opioids and/or local anesthetics into the epidural space and can be used to manage pain in equine patients on a short-term (hours to days) or long-term (weeks) basis (**Table 2**). For longer term management, the placement of a caudal epidural catheter can be beneficial for repeated administration of analgesic drugs.

Table 2
Dose and volume recommendations for analgesic drugs epidurally delivered used for pain management in horses with laminitis

Drug	Volume	Duration
Caudal epidurally administered		
Xylazine 0.18 mg/kg + morphine 0.2 mg/kg	qs 0.1–0.2 mL/kg bwt	8–12 h
Cervical epidurally administered		
Morphine 0.1 mg/kg	qs 0.01 mL/kg bwt[81]	12 h

Abbreviations: bwt, body weight; qs, at hour of sleep.

The placement of caudal epidural catheters in horses for the long-term management of moderate to severe pain showed good results and has been described since the early 1980s.[71] A retrospective study looking at outcome in 50 cases of caudal epidural catheter placement in horses indicated that epidural catheterization can be used successfully for the repeated epidural delivery of analgesics and anesthetics in horses with various clinical conditions. Complications associated with epidural catheters or epidural drug administration were infrequent and transient in this study.[72]

The recommended caudal epidural protocols are not only dose but also volume dependent regarding the localization of pain and the size of the horse. Morphine is commonly used and often combined with an α-2 agonist such as xylazine to increase duration of action from 8 to 10 hours to 12 to 16 hours.[73,74] Although pelvic limb analgesia is often reliably achieved using a dose of 0.1 to 0.2 mg/kg morphine in an injected volume of 0.05 to 0.10 mL/kg bodyweight, the analgesic efficacy of caudal epidurally administered morphine is less reliable and requires higher injectate volumes of up to 0.2 mL/kg bodyweight in cases with moderate to severe thoracic limb pain.

Cervical Epidural Catheter

Recently, the use of a new epidural analgesic technique was described. Cervical epidural analgesia has been used in human medicine to treat neck disease and pain.[75] In horses, the use of caudal epidural analgesia is more established and described, but particularly thoracic limb pain treatment can be challenging with caudal epidural analgesia.

Hurcombe and colleagues[76] described the placement of cervical epidural and intrathecal catheters in healthy horses. This technique requires more advanced equipment, such as ultrasound and radiography, to confirm the anatomic location of the catheters. However, all horses tolerated the catheter placement well for the duration of the study, with no signs of discomfort, and cerebrospinal fluid parameters did not change over the study period. Ongoing research is currently evaluating the antinociceptive effects of cervical epidural morphine in horses and the preliminary results are encouraging with morphine providing long-lasting and reliable antinociception. Low volumes and dosages of morphine (0.10 mg/kg morphine qs to 0.01 mL/kg) confirmed effective and long-lasting analgesia of the thoracic limb for up to 16 hours.

Long-term Local Blocks

One safe way to provide analgesia of the distal limb is the use of local anesthetic drugs and nerve blocks. The main limitation for nerve blocks is often the relatively short duration of action of only a few hours for most local anesthetic drugs, making repeated injection necessary for longer lasting analgesia and anesthesia. Bupivacaine is one of the longest-acting local anesthetic drugs, but its duration of action is generally considered to be 6 to 8 hours.[77] An extended-release formulation of the local anesthetic bupivacaine (Exparel; Pacira Pharmaceuticals) became available for humans in 2011, and its counterpart (Nocita; Elanco) was recently approved for use in dogs and cats. A pilot study in small animals showed that a single injection of this bupivacaine formulation provides analgesia for up to 72 hours.[78] This drug may, therefore, have clinical application in addressing the unmet need for effective and long-lasting local analgesia in horses.

Studies in horses, however, showed mixed results. In a recently published study, the perineural injection of liposomal bupivacaine meaningfully increased the mechanical nociceptive threshold of the digit but lasted only for 30 minutes to 4 hours after injection.[79] The reasons for the differences in duration between small animals and horses remain unclear.

Another way for long-term local blockage is the placement of perineural catheters. Continuous peripheral nerve block is a method that has long been used with good success in human medicine to treat patients suffering from severe extremity pain. The method entails the continuous infusion of local anesthetics via catheters placed alongside peripheral nerves and has been shown to provide better pain control with fewer side effects than systemic analgesics, to improve functional recovery, and to shorten hospital stay. A recent article described a technique for placing continuous peripheral nerve block catheters adjacent to palmar nerves in horses and to evaluate the effect of low-volume local anesthetic infusion on nociception in the distal equine thoracic limb.[80] Despite the successful placement of these catheters and their efficacy to prevent response to noxious stimuli, the authors further reported significant limb swelling and edema formation within 1 to 2 days during lidocaine or mepivacaine infusion. At this point, the use of these catheters is therefore clinically limited.

SUMMARY

One of the greatest challenges in managing laminitis in horses remains the control of pain. Currently, the best analgesic approach is multimodal with a combination of systemic protocols including NSAIDs, opioids and/or constant rate infusions of α-2 agonists, ketamine, and lidocaine. Newer literature indicates that the use of amitriptyline and soluble epoxide hydrolase inhibitor might be beneficial. Clinically evidenced-based, large studies are needed to demonstrate if they have a place in laminitis pain management.

The systemic pain control can be combined with local techniques such as long-lasting local anesthetics or various techniques of epidural catheterization that allows for administration of potent analgesic therapy with a lower risk of negative side effects.

CLINICS CARE POINTS

- NSAIDs are still the foundation for successful management of foot pain.
- Newer α-2 agonists such as dexmedetomidine may not only provide strong analgesia, but also have tissue-protective effects.
- Epidural analgesia as well as caudal and cervical epidural catheters offer a new clinical option for effective analgesia with less drug-related side effects.

DISCLOSURE

The authors have nothing to disclose.

REFERENCES

1. Knights KM, Mangoni AA, Miners JO. Defining the COX inhibitor selectivity of NSAIDs: implications for understanding toxicity. Expert Rev Clin Pharmacol 2010;3:769–76.
2. Hinz B, Cheremina O, Brune K. Acetaminophen (paracetamol) is a selective cyclooxygenase-2 inhibitor in man. FASEB J 2008;22:383–90.
3. Fowler CJ. The contribution of cyclooxygenase-2 to endocannabinoid metabolism and action. Br J Pharmacol 2007;152:594–601.
4. Rouzer CA, Marnett LJ. Non-redundant functions of cyclooxygenases: oxygenation of endocannabinoids. J Biol Chem 2008;283:8065–9.
5. Hamza M, Dionne RA. Mechanisms of non-opioid analgesics beyond cyclooxygenase enzyme inhibition. Curr Mol Pharmacol 2009;2:1–14.
6. Sumano Lopez H, Hoyos Sepulveda ML, Brumbaugh GW. Pharmacologic and alternative therapies for the horse with chronic laminitis. Vet Clin North Am Equine Pract 1999;15:495–516.
7. Belknap JK. Treatment of the acute laminitis case. In: Large animal proceedings of the North American Veterinary Conference. Orlando (FL); January 7-11, 2006: 76–80.
8. Moore RM. Evidence-based treatment for laminitis - what works? J Equine Vet Sci 2008;28:176–9.
9. Clark JO, Clark TP. Analgesia. Vet Clin North Am Equine Pract 1999;15:705–23.
10. Moyer W, Schumacher J, Schumacher J, et al. Are drugs effective treatment for horses with acute laminitis? In: Proceedings of the 54th Annual Convention of the American association of equine Practioners, San Diego (CA); January 7-11, 2008: 337–340.
11. Simon LS. Biology and toxic effects of nonsteroidal anti-inflammatory drugs. Curr Opin Rheumatol 1998;10:153–8.
12. Blikslager A. Role of NSAIDs in the management of pain in horses. In: Proceedings of the American association of equine practitioners focus meeting. Raleigh (NC); January 7-11, 2009: 218–223.
13. Divers TJ. COX inhibitors: making the best choice for the laminitic case. J Equine Vet Sci 2008;28:367–9.
14. Urdaneta A, Siso A, Urdaneta B, et al. Lack of correlation between the central anti-nociceptive and peripheral anti-inflammatory effects of selective COX-2 inhibitor parecoxib. Brain Res Bull 2009;80:56–61.
15. Bovill JG. Mechanisms of actions of opioids and non-steroidal anti-inflammatory drugs. Eur J Anaesthesiol 1997;14:9–15.
16. Surratt CK, Johnson PS, Moriwaki A, et al. µ opiate receptor. Charged transmembrane domain amino acids are critical for agonist recognition and intrinsic activity. J Biol Chem 1994;269:20548–53.
17. McFadzean DF. The ionic mechanisms underlying opioid actions. Neuropeptides 1988;11:173–80.
18. Crain SM, Shen KF. Opioids can evoke direct receptor-mediated excitatory effects on sensory neurons. Trends Pharmacol Sci 1990;11:77–81.
19. De Leon-Cassola OA, Lema MJ. Postoperative epidural opioid analgesia: what are the choices? Anesth Analg 1996;83:867–75.
20. Ferreira SH, Nakamura M. II. Prostaglandin hyperalgesia: the peripheral analgesic activity of morphine, enkephalins and opioid antagonists. Prostaglandins 1979;18:191–200.

21. Reid JL. Central alpha 2 receptors and the regulation of blood pressure in humans. J Cardiovasc Pharmacol 1985;7(Suppl 8):S45–50.

22. Brosda J, Jantschak F, Pertz HH. α2-Adrenoceptors are targets for antipsychotic drugs. Psychopharmacology (Berl) 2014;231:801–12.

23. Gyires K, Zádori ZS, Török T, et al. Alpha(2)-Adrenoceptor subtypes-mediated physiological, pharmacological actions. Neurochem Int 2009;55:447–53.

24. Asano T, Dohi S, Ohta S, et al. Antinociception by epidural and systemic alpha(2)-adrenoceptor agonists and their binding affinity in rat spinal cord and brain. Anesth Analg 2000;90:400–40.

25. Murry CE, Jennings RB, Reimer KA. Preconditioning with ischemia: a delay of lethal cell injury in ischemic myocardium. Circulation 1986;74:1124–36.

26. König KS, Verhaar N, Hopster K, et al. Ischaemic preconditioning and pharmacological preconditioning with dexmedetomidine in an equine model of small intestinal ischaemia-reperfusion. PLoS One 2020;15:e0224720.

27. VanderBroek AR, Engiles JB, Kästner SBR, et al. Protective effects of dexmedetomidine on small intestinal ischaemia-reperfusion injury in horses. Equine Vet J 2021;53:569–78.

28. Attal N, Cruccu G, Baron R, et al. EFNS guidelines on the pharmacological treatment of neuropathic pain: 2010 revision. Eur J Neurol 2010;17:1113–88.

29. Moulin DE, Clark AJ, Gilron I, et al. Pharmacological management of chronic neuropathic pain - consensus statement and guidelines from the Canadian Pain Society. Pain Res Manag 2007;12:13–21.

30. Finnerup NB, Attal N, Haroutounian S, et al. Pharmacotherapy for neuropathic pain in adults: a systematic review and meta-analysis. Lancet Neurol 2015;14:162–73.

31. Terry RL, McDonnell SM, Van Eps AW, et al. Pharmacokinetic profile and behavioral effects of gabapentin in the horse. J Vet Pharmacol Ther 2010;33:485–94.

32. Davis JL, Posner LP, Elce Y. Gabapentin for the treatment of neuropathic pain in a pregnant horse. J Am Vet Med Assoc 2007;231:755–8.

33. Young JM, Schoonover MJ, Kembel SL, et al. Efficacy of orally administered gabapentin in horses with chronic thoracic limb lameness. Vet Anaesth Analg 2020;47:259–66.

34. Mion G, Villevieille T. Ketamine pharmacology: an update (pharmacodynamics and molecular aspects, recent findings). CNS Neurosci Ther 2013;19:370–80.

35. Peltoniemi MA, Hagelberg NM, Olkkola KT, et al. Ketamine: a review of clinical pharmacokinetics and pharmacodynamics in anesthesia and pain therapy. Clin Pharmacokinet 2016;55:1059–77.

36. Lu W, Wang L, Wo C, et al. Ketamine attenuates osteoarthritis of the knee via modulation of inflammatory responses in a rabbit model. Mol Med Rep 2016;13:5013–20.

37. Dale O, Somogyi AA, Li Y, et al. Does intraoperative ketamine attenuate inflammatory reactivity following surgery? A systematic review and meta-analysis. Anesth Analg 2012;115:934–43.

38. Müller TM, Hopster K, Bienert-Zeit A, et al. Effect of butorphanol, midazolam or ketamine on romifidine based sedation in horses during standing cheek tooth removal. BMC Vet Res 2017;13:381.

39. Fielding CL, Brumbaugh GW, Matthews NS, et al. Pharmacokinetics and clinical effects of a subanesthetic continuous rate infusion of ketamine in awake horses. Am J Vet Res 2006;67:1484–90.

40. Guedes AG, Matthews NS, Hood DM. Effect of ketamine hydrochloride on the analgesic effects of tramadol hydrochloride in horses with signs of chronic laminitis-associated pain. Am J Vet Res 2012;73:610–9.

41. Hara M, Kai Y, Ikemoto Y. Local anesthetics reduce the inhibitory neurotransmitter-induced current in dissociated hippocampal neurons of the rat. Eur J Pharmacol 1995;283:83–9.

42. Ye JH, Ren J, Krnjevic K, et al. Cocaine and lidocaine have additive inhibitory effects on the GABAA current of acutely dissociated hippocampal pyramidal neurons. Brain Res 1999;821:26–32.

43. Sugimoto M, Uchida I, Fukami S, et al. The alpha and gamma subunit-dependent effects of local anesthetics on recombinant GABA(A) receptors. Eur J Pharmacol 2000;401:329–37.

44. Todorov AA, Kolchev CB, Todorov AB. Tiagabine and gabapentin for the management of chronic pain. Clin J Pain 2005;21:358–61.

45. Sommer C, Leinders M, Uceyler N. Inflammation in the pathophysiology of neuropathic pain. Pain 2018;159:595–602.

46. Giddon DB, Lindhe J. In vivo quantitation of local anesthetic suppression of leukocyte adherence. Am J Pathol 1972;68:327–38.

47. MacGregor RR, Thorner RE, Wright DM. Lidocaine inhibits granulocyte adherence and prevents granulocyte delivery to inflammatory sites. Blood 1980;56:203–9.

48. Kanbara T, Tomoda MK, Sato EF, et al. Lidocaine inhibits priming and protein tyrosine phosphorylation of human peripheral neutrophils. Biochem Pharmacol 1993;45:1593–8.

49. Hollmann MW, Gross A, Jelacin N, et al. Local anesthetic effects on priming and activation of human neutrophils. Anesthesiology 2001;95:113–22.

50. Mikawa K, Maekawa N, Nishina K, et al. Effect of lidocaine pretreatment on endotoxin-induced lung injury in rabbits. Anesthesiology 1994;81:689–99.

51. Nishina K, Mikawa K, Maekawa N, et al. Does early posttreatment with lidocaine attenuate endotoxin-induced acute injury in rabbits? Anesthesiology 1995;83:169–77.

52. Taniguchi T, Shibata K, Yamamoto K, et al. Effects of lidocaine administration on hemodynamics and cytokine responses to endotoxemia in rabbits. Crit Care Med 2000;28:755–9.

53. Kiyonari Y, Nishina K, Mikawa K, et al. Lidocaine attenuates acute lung injury induced by a combination of phospholipase A2 and trypsin. Crit Care Med 2000;28:484–9.

54. Flondor M, Listle H, Kemming GI, et al. Effect of inhaled and intravenous lidocaine on inflammatory reaction in endotoxaemic rats. Eur J Anaesthesiol 2010;27:53–60.

55. Shiga M, Nishina K, Mikawa K, et al. The effects of lidocaine on nitric oxide production from an activated murine macrophage cell line. Anesth Analg 2001;92:128–33.

56. Huang YH, Tsai PS, Kai YF, et al. Lidocaine inhibition of inducible nitric oxide synthase and cationic amino acid transporter-2 transcription in activated murine macrophages may involve voltage-sensitive $Na+$ channel. Anesth Analg 2006;102:1739–44.

57. Takaishi K, Kitahata H, Kawahito S. Local anesthetics inhibit nitric oxide production and L-arginine uptake in cultured bovine aortic endothelial cells. Eur J Pharmacol 2013;704:58–63.

58. Piegeler T, Votta-Velis EG, Bakhshi FR, et al. Endothelial barrier protection by local anesthetics: ropivacaine and lidocaine block tumor necrosis factor-alpha-induced endothelial cell Src activation. Anesthesiology 2014;120:1414–28.

59. Paoli F, Darcourt G, Cossa P. Preliminary note on the action of imipramine in painful states. Rev Neurol 1960;102:503–4.

60. Max MB, Culnane M, Schafer SC, et al. Amitriptyline relieves diabetic neuropathy pain in patients with normal or depressed mood. Neurology 1987;37:589–96.

61. Mico JA, Ardid D, Berrocoso E, et al. Antidepressants and pain. Trends Pharmacol Sci 2006;27:348–54.

62. Watson CP, Chipman M, Reed K, et al. Amitriptyline versus maprotiline in postherpetic neuralgia: a randomized, double-blind, crossover trial. Pain 1992;48:29–36.

63. Wagner K, Inceoglu B, Hammoc BD. Soluble epoxide hydrolase inhibition, epoxygenated fatty acids and nociception. Prostaglandins Other Lipid Mediat 2011a; 96:76–83.

64. Wagner K, Inceoglu B, Hammoc BD. Epoxygenated fatty acids and soluble epoxide hydrolase inhibition: novel mediators of pain reduction. J Agric Food Chem 2011b;59:2816–24.

65. Morisseau C, Inceoglu B, Schmelzer K, et al. Naturally occurring monoepoxides of eicosapentaenoic acid and docosahexaenoic acid are bioactive antihyperalgesic lipids. J Lipid Res 2010;51:3481–90.

66. Inceoglu B, Jinks SL, Ulu A, et al. Soluble epoxide hydrolase and epoxyeicosatrienoic acids modulate two distinct analgesic pathways. Proc Natl Acad Sci 2008;105:18901–6.

67. Terashvili M, Tseng LF, Wu HE, et al. Antinociception produced by 14,15-epoxyeicosatrienoic acid is mediated by the activation of beta-endorphin and met-enkephalin in the rat ventrolateral periaqueductal gray. J Pharmacol Exp Ther 2008;326:614–22.

68. Inceoglu B, Wagner KM, Yang J, et al. Acute augmentation of epoxygenated fatty acid levels rapidly reduces pain-related behavior in a rat model of type I diabetes. Proc Natl Acad Sci 2012;109:11390–5.

69. Guedes AG, Morisseau C, Sole A, et al. Use of a soluble epoxide hydrolase inhibitor as an adjunctive analgesic in a horse with laminitis. Vet Anaesth Analg 2013; 40:440–8.

70. Jones E, Vinuela-Fernandez I, Eager RA, et al. Neuropathic changes in equine laminitis pain. Pain 2007;132:321–31.

71. Green EM, Cooper RC. Continuous caudal epidural anesthesia in the horse. J Am Vet Med Assoc 1984;184:971–4.

72. Martin CA, Kerr CL, Pearce SG, et al. Outcome of epidural catheterization for delivery of analgesics in horses: 43 cases (1998-2001). J Am Vet Med Assoc 2003; 222:1394–8.

73. Natalini CC, Robinson EP. Evaluation of the analgesic effects of epidurally administered morphine, alfentanil, butorphanol, tramadol, and U50488H in horses. Am J Vet Res 2000;61:1579–86.

74. Robinson EP, Natalini CC. Epidural anesthesia and analgesia in horses. Vet Clin North Am Equine Pract 2002;18:61–82.

75. Bromage PR, Bramwell RS, Catchlove RF, et al. Peridurography with metrizamide: animal and human studies. Radiology 1978;128:123–6.

76. Hurcombe SD, Morris TB, VanderBroek AR, et al. Cervical Epidural and Subarachnoid Catheter Placement in Standing Adult Horses. Front Vet Sci 2020; 7:232.

77. Lerche P, Aarnes TK, Covey-Crump G, et al. Handbook of small animal Regional Anesthesia and analgesia techniques. Chichester, West Sussex, UK: John Wiley & Sons; 2016. p. 10–9.
78. Lascelles BDX, Rausch-Derra LC, Wofford JA, et al. Pilot, randomized, placebo-controlled clinical field study to evaluate the effectiveness of bupivacaine liposome injectable suspension for the provision of post-surgical analgesia in dogs undergoing stifle surgery. BMC Vet Res 2016;12:168.
79. McCracken MJ, Schumacher J, Doherty TJ, et al. Efficacy and duration of effect for liposomal bupivacaine when administered perineurally to the palmar digital nerves of horses. Am J Vet Res 2020;81:400–5.
80. Driessen B, Scandella M, Zarucco L. Development of a technique for continuous perineural blockade of the palmar nerves in the distal equine thoracic limb. Vet Anaesth Analg 2008;35:432–48.
81. Watkins AR, Hopster K, Levine D, et al. Cervical epidural catheter placement for pain management of forelimb superficial digital flexor muscle tear in a Quarter Horse gelding: case report. Front Vet Sci. 12

Imaging the Equine Foot

Aitor Gallastegui, LV, MSc

KEYWORDS

- Diagnostic imaging • Equine • Foot • Current advances

KEY POINTS

- Current radiographic techniques applied to the equine foot allow more accurate diagnoses and reduce radiation exposure.
- PET–computed tomography (CT) allows detection of active foot lesion on the standing horse with high sensitivity and possibly earlier than other diagnostic imaging modalities.
- CT can be acquired safely in the standing horse, increasing the possibilities and safety of this modality in general equine practice. The intraoperative use of CT is discussed.
- High-field magnetic resonance imaging and contrast magnetic resonance imaging have the potential to improve the evaluation of cartilage, ligaments, and pathologies of the hoof lamina.

Diagnostic imaging remains one of the most important diagnostic tools used in the assessment, diagnosis, and monitoring of injuries to the equine foot. As technology and knowledge improve, veterinarians can overcome many of the challenges inherent to the identification of multiple anatomic structures and their superimposition in the hoof. This article reviews the most significant advances in imaging of the foot that have occurred over the past 5 years and discusses some of the most current and future advances that are to come.

DIGITAL RADIOLOGY

Radiology remains the diagnostic modality used most frequently for imaging the foot in both ambulatory and referral practices. Its low cost, portability, and the improved image quality provided by the digital transformation of the radiology systems make it an essential and extremely useful first-hand tool for imaging the foot in horses. In addition, digital images allow fast transmission of the studies via the Internet for consultation with radiologists for a second opinion, providing improved patient care for all horses, regardless of their location.

Over the past half decade, the radiographic technique for the foot has improved, as it has been learned that centering the x-ray beam on the foot/floor interphase works

Small Animal Clinical Sciences, University of Florida, 2015 Southwest 16th Avenue, Gainesville, FL 32608, USA
E-mail address: aitorgallastegui@ufl.edu

Vet Clin Equine 37 (2021) 563–579
https://doi.org/10.1016/j.cveq.2021.07.003
0749-0739/21/© 2021 Elsevier Inc. All rights reserved.

vetequine.theclinics.com

best for measuring the palmar angle,[1] that unipedal stance has a negative effect on radiographic anatomic obliquity,[2] and that obliquity on lateromedial radiographs has a negative effect on the assessment of distal interphalangeal effusion or capsular thickening.[3] In addition, as knowledge in cross-sectional imaging of the foot improves, so does the accuracy of the radiographic diagnoses. Improvement of the radiographic protocols also has helped reduce the radiation exposure and the work time associated with taking radiographs. As such, it has been learned that taking a single diagnostic quality dorsoproximal-palmarodistal oblique radiograph produces diagnostic images of both the distal phalanx and the navicular bone, when using appropriate postprocessing and manipulation.[4] The principles of using radiographs for pathologic trimming and shoeing were recently described by Redden and Smith.[5]

Reviews on the radiographic examination of the foot were described by Dyson[6] and Redden[7]. Many of these descriptions, however, are based on film or early digital radiographic technology, and many veterinarians might consider them obsolete, considering how much the image quality has improved since their original publication. The advancements in technology and image quality result in increased identification of radiographic variations, many of which not always are associated with pathology. Therefore, readers should recognize that the image interpretation skills need to advance in parallel with technology advances.

Some of the most recently recognized normal variations include the occasional identification of sharp bony margins at the dorsal aspect of the distal interphalangeal joint, which may resemble osteophyte formation. In these cases, the acquisition of additional radiographs, such as the dorso-60°proximo45°-lateral-palmarodistomedial and the dorso-60°proximo45°-medial-palmarodistolateral oblique projections might be recommended to highlight the dorsomedial and dorsolateral articular margins, and confirm or rule out the presence of osteoarthrosis.[8]

In the navicular bone, a crescent lucency seen at the flexor crest on the palmaro-45°proximal-palmarodistal oblique projection, represents a normal region of noncompact bone between a reinforcement line of the cancellous bone and the flexor cortex.[9] This lucency, however, often is misread by less experienced observers or, in more ill-defined cases, as lysis of the flexor cortex, which is known to carry a poor prognosis.[10] Acquiring more shallow palmaroproximal-palmarodistal oblique projections (ie, 35°–45° to the horizontal plane) improves the accuracy of detection and characterization of lysis at the flexor cortex of the navicular bone (**Fig. 1**).[11] In this study, observers of all levels of experience performed more uniformly identifying lysis and assessing its severity when they had multiple skyline projections available for review. Overall, the use of multiple views to detect flexor cortical lysis in the navicular bone resulted in improvement of the sensitivity and interobserver agreement but resulted in reduction of specificity.

A recent study identified regions of new bone formation in the distal and proximal phalanges in association with extensive ossification of the ungual cartilages.[12] This new bone formation was more common when an ossification grade greater than or equal to 4 of the ungual cartilages was present. Increasing age was a reduced risk factor for development of new bone formation on the distal phalanx but a risk factor for the presence of new bone formation on the proximal phalanx. According to earlier publications, ossification of the ungular cartilages could be a cause of pain and lameness and is examined best on dorsopalmar and dorsolateral-palmaromedial or dorsomedial-palmarolateral oblique radiographic projections. Therefore, identification of new bone formation at these sites in horses with lameness that does not respond to standard medical management may suggest the need for advanced imaging, such as magnetic resonance imaging (MRI) or PET.

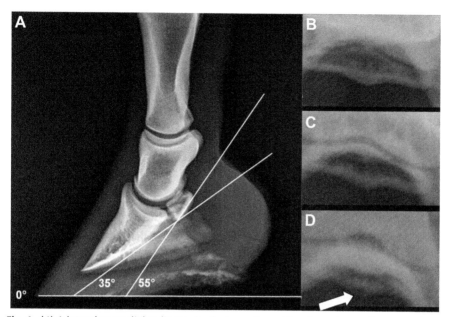

Fig. 1. (*A*) A lateral to medial radiograph of a horse in position to make a palmaroproximal-palmarodistal oblique (navicular skyline) radiograph. Angles of incidence have been measured in reference to the horizontal (35° and 55°), with lines extended to demonstrate proposed beam trajectory. Note how a flatter angle of incidence (35°) makes the beam tangential to the more distal portion of the navicular bone in contrast to the more traditional 55° angle that would make the beam tangential to the more proximal portion of the navicular bone. (*B–D*) Palmaroproximal-palmarodistal oblique (navicular skyline) radiographs at known beam angles ([*B*] 55°, [*C*] 45°, and [*D*] 35°) demonstrating mild to moderate lysis (*arrow*). Note how the appearance of the distally located flexor cortical lysis becomes more apparent with a flatter angle of incidence. (*Adapted from*[11] with permission.)

Current studies have identified an association between a negative or a neutral plantar distal phalanx angle and pelvic limb lameness. As expected, these angles are measured best on standing lateromedial radiographs of the foot. A study in a UK population of horses identified horses with pelvic limb lameness, which was localized to the stifle primarily, were more likely to have a negative plantar distal phalanx angle.[13] An earlier study identified that horses with lameness localized to the distal tarsus and proximal metatarsus, but not to the stifle, were more likely to have a negative or neutral plantar distal phalanx angle.[14] The disagreement on the correlation between abnormal plantar angles and the location of the lameness might reflect differences in the sampled populations. It still is unknown, however, whether lameness localized to these regions was the result of a negative or neutral plantar distal phalanx angle or vice versa.

Laminitis remains one of the most common pathologies for which radiographs of the foot are acquired. A study showed no benefit of using a lead marker on the dorsal hoof wall for measurements when using digital radiography.[15] Another recent study examined the ratio of the hoof distal phalanx distance to the length of the palmar aspect of the distal phalanx (named the HDPD ratio) in a large population of horses at proximal, mid, and distal levels.[16] Although the mean HDPD ratio was in agreement with earlier studies (0.25 ± 0.03), there was considerable variation in the relative proximal, mid, and distal measurements of the HDPD within and among horses. Although it was not statistically significant, horses with distal measurements larger than the proximal measurements had been shod less recently, suggesting that the interval since the last trimming and shoeing might account for some of the variability seen between the measurements at different levels. In horses with HDPD ratios greater than 0.25, modeling (slipper formation) of the toe and/or new bone formation at the dorsal aspect of the distal phalanx was seen frequently. Although some of these changes can be seen with other pathologies, upon identification of HDPD ratios greater than 0.25, the investigators recommended careful examination of the foot for other supporting evidence of lamellar pathology, giving thought to testing for equine metabolic syndrome and/ or pituitary pars intermedia dysfunction and considering appropriate management for chronic laminitis. In addition, given the small variation of these ratios among the thoracic limbs, even negligible increases in the ratio on 1 foot, compared with the contralateral, may suggest lamellar pathology and should not be ignored. Of the 415 feet examined (from 279 horses with foot pain and no known history of laminitis or clinical signs of acute laminitis), however, 42.2% had an HDPD ratio greater than 0.25.

Positive contrast venography has become an important tool for the assessment of areas of vascular compression or injury within the foot and is used most frequently on laminitic patients, with a special focus on the assessment of the circumflex vessels and the lamellar circumflex junction (**Fig. 2**A, B).[17] Positive contrast venography also can be used to evaluate nonlaminitic foot disease and the inclusion of the 60°-dorsoproximo-palmarodistal oblique projection allowed for more accurate localization of vascular disturbances of the digit (**Fig. 2**C).[18] Venograms provide information regarding the mechanical forces that act in association with the foot pathology, which then can be altered with trimming, shoeing, and surgery, resulting in improvement of patient comfort and prognosis. Contrast venograms are possible to perform as an ambulatory service. A current limitation of venograms is the lack of studies that have identified specific long-term radiographic prognostic indicators.

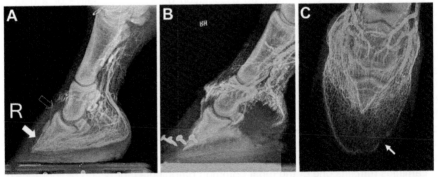

Fig. 2. (*A*) A lateromedial digital venogram image with an irregular filling defect on the coronary plexus (*black arrow*) and contrast extravasation along the dorsal sublamellar plexus (*white arrow*) in a horse with acute laminitis. (*B*) Two-week recheck lateromedial digital venogram on the same horse as (*B*) with progressive palmar rotation of the distal phalanx and severe vascular compromise. (*C*) A dorsoproximo-palmarodistal digital venogram image with filling defects of the circumflex vessels at the dorsomedial solar margin (*arrow*), associated with a nonaggressive lytic lesion secondary to a keratoma.

ULTRASONOGRAPHY

Despite ultrasonography being the second most used imaging modality in equine musculoskeletal disease, ultrasonography of the foot is limited by the hoof capsule, which does not allow the transmission of the ultrasound beam and imaging of the structures contained within it. Only 2 ultrasonographic windows allow limited examination of some of the structures of the foot:

- The heel bulb approach allows visualization of the more distal portion of the deep digital flexor tendon (DDFT) over the middle phalanx, the collateral sesamoidean ligament, the proximal margin of the navicular bone, the proximal recess of the distal interphalangeal joint, the navicular bursa, and the palmar/plantar aspect of the middle phalanx.
- The transcuneal approach allows visualization of the insertion of the DDFT, the plantar/palmar border of the navicular bone, the impar ligament, the navicular bursa, the distal recess of the distal interphalangeal joint, and a portion of distal phalanx. This approach, however, requires extensive preparation of the hoof to allow optimal transmission of the ultrasound beam through the sole and, therefore, is time consuming and used infrequently.

Compared with MRI, ultrasound was sensitive for evaluation of moderate to severe tears of the DDFT at the proximal recess of the navicular bursa but can overestimate or underestimate the soft tissue changes, whereas distal lesions in the DDFT might be missed with the heel bulb approach. Ultrasound sensitivity also increased with increased severity of tears along the dorsal margin of the DDFT.[19] Conversely, MRI and ultrasound showed the same accuracy (87.5%) at detecting flexor adhesions within the hoof.[20]

NUCLEAR MEDICINE

Nuclear scintigraphy has been used extensively in equine orthopedic imaging for approximately 40 years, and for a long time many private practices and most veterinary colleges had gamma cameras. The most unique characteristic of scintigraphy is its ability to identify metabolically active and, therefore, clinically relevant, lesions. Although skeletal scintigraphy is sensitive, it is relatively nonspecific for determining a specific etiology. Despite that image quality has improved significantly with technology advances, the spatial resolution of bone scintigraphy is limited; therefore, it requires correlation of the findings with other modalities, primarily radiology and more recently computed tomography (CT) and MRI. A recent study demonstrated that nuclear scintigraphy alone is unlikely to lead to a full and correct diagnosis of the cause of lameness or poor performance in horses when used as an isolated screening tool, with up to 64.5% false-negative results.[21]

Recently a new modality has emerged in the field of equine nuclear imaging, and that is the PET. PET is a cross-sectional functional imaging modality and is extensively used in human oncologic imaging and neuroimaging for which ^{18}F-fluorodeoxyglucose (^{18}F-FDG) is the radiopharmaceutical used most frequently. ^{18}F-FDG is a radioactive glucose that concentrates in areas of increased metabolic activity, such as tumors. In PET, the detectors are arranged in a ring, similar to the arrangement of receptors in CT gantries. This arrangement allows identification of areas of uptake within a 3-dimensional (3-D) space, avoiding the superimposition artifact present on 2-dimensional radiographic or scintigraphic studies and resulting in improved spatial resolution.

In orthopedic imaging, ^{18}F-sodium fluoride (^{18}F-NaF) is the radiopharmaceutical of choice. Fluoride from ^{18}F-NaF is trapped at the exposed hydroxyapatite bone matrix, in a similar way to ^{99m}-technetium methyl diphosphonate (^{99m}Tc-MDP), which is the radiopharmaceutical used in nuclear scintigraphy. The benefits of PET over bone scan scintigraphy include: higher spatial resolution, cross-sectional imaging that eliminates the superimposition of anatomic structures, more accurate quantification, small size, and in some instances portability.[22,23] The functional information provided by PET can be improved further by fussing the images obtained in PET scans with images acquired with CT or MRI. Conventional PET scanners normally are coupled to a CT gantry conforming what is known as a PET-CT scanner. Provided the appropriate software is available, images obtained with independent PET, CT, and/or MRI scanners can be fused, although the efficiency of this process is reduced compared with the efficiency of the combined systems.

The use of PET scanners in imaging of the equine orthopedic patient was pioneered by Dr Spriet at the University of California, Davis. Dr Spriet started using portable PET scanners on horses under general anesthesia in 2015 and recently developed and validated an equine specific standing portable open PET ring scanner (**Fig. 3**).[24,25] Besides having access to the equipment for a PET scanner, however, a nearby source of the appropriate radiopharmaceutical is needed. The reduced half-life of ^{18}F-NaF (109.7 min compared with the approximately 6 h of ^{9m}Tc) limits the location of the practices that can offer this imaging modality. A short half-life results in a reduction of the hospitalization time required for completing the clearance of the patients undergoing a nuclear study. Therefore, these patients can be discharged as early as the same day the PET study is performed.

To date, equine PET has proved to be a simple procedure, with radiation doses similar to those of regular equine scintigraphy[26] and PET is able to detect focal ^{18}F-NaF uptake in areas where other imaging modalities, such as CT, standing scintigraphy, and standing MRI, do not always identify abnormalities (**Fig. 4**). Such lesions are described at ligamentous attachments, the subchondral compact bone plate, the flexor cortex of the navicular bone, and the DDFT.[26–29] In addition, the lack of radiopharmaceutical uptake at sites of abnormal bone proliferation or fragmentation,

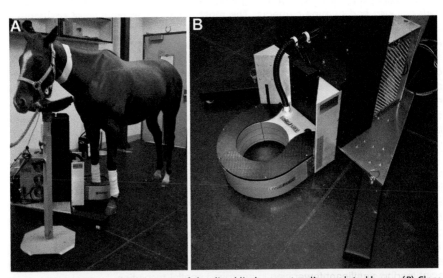

Fig. 3. (A) Acquisition of PET images of the distal limb on a standing sedated horse. (B) Close look at the open ring conformation of MILE-PET(R) (Longmile, Veterinary Imaging, 12156 Parklawn Drive, Rockville, MD 20852, USA) standing equine PET scanner, with permission. (*Courtesy of* Dr. Mathieu Spriet from the University of California, Davis.)

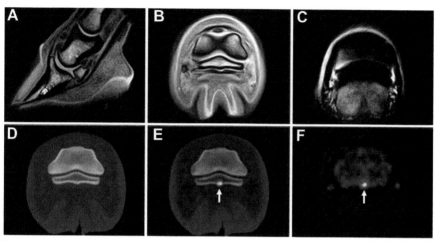

Fig. 4. MRI images in sagittal T1-weighted (*A*), transverse T1-weighted (*B*), and transverse STIR (*C*) planes and sequences of a 3-year-old American quarter horse mare with lameness localized to the foot. (*D*) CT transverse image of the foot in bone algorithm on the same horse. Fused ^{18}F-NaF PET/CT (*E*) and ^{18}F-NaF PET (*F*) of the same horse. Although no abnormalities are detected on MRI and CT, PET detects marked focal increased ^{18}F-NaF uptake at the sagittal ridge of the flexor cortex (*arrows*). This is considered an early sign of degenerative changes of the navicular bone. (*Courtesy of* Dr. Mathieu Spriet from the University of California, Davis.)

suggests that PET is capable of distinguishing between active and inactive lesions.[26] Despite the toe and central regions of the distal phalanx having higher uptake than other areas within the bone,[30] PET may be able to differentiate between acute and chronic cases of laminitis based on the distribution of areas of maximal standardized uptake values.[31]

COMPUTED TOMOGRAPHY

Performing a CT study of the foot has been available for equine patients since CT-coupled large animal tables became available, and the CT anatomy of the equine foot is well described elsewhere.[32] The need for general anesthesia, however, has limited its use primarily to the surgical management of third phalanx fractures, fractures of the navicular bone, and keratomas.[33–35]

In the operating room, CT scanners can be coupled with surgery navigation systems, which operate together with cameras tracking the surgical instruments. These systems constitute the basis of computer-assisted orthopedic surgery (CAOS) and provide the surgeon with simultaneous real-time information on the position and orientation of the instruments in relation to the surgical anatomy. This technology can improve surgical accuracy and better patient outcomes, particularly in complex orthopedic cases.[36] In a recent study, 3-D–assisted surgery was compared with conservative methods in the management of type III fractures of the distal phalanx, and, although there was no effect on time to recovery between the 2 groups, surgical treatment lead to significant fewer cases of distal interphalangeal osteoarthrosis as determined by subjective radiographic evaluation.[37]

The limitations of CT-CAOS include the need for a dedicated surgical CT scanner, increased radiation exposure, and a potential need for separate teams that plan or execute the surgeries in order to optimize workflow and time efficiency.[33] The use of portable CT units (**Fig. 5**) or the development of multifunctional CT rooms (**Fig. 6A**) might be able to relieve some of the economical and operational constraints on the intraoperative use of CT scanners. The use of commercially available aiming devices in combination with CT allowed precision fixation of all third phalanx leading to favorable outcome in 13 of 14 horses (**Fig. 6B, C**).[38] In addition, improved surgical protocols and the addition of surgical navigation systems may limit the radiation doses compared to the use of CT alone. Although the dose to the patient can be a concern for some applications, particularly in human pediatric spinal surgery, it appears that although the dose to the patient remains similar, the use of intraoperative CT decreases the amount of radiation to the surgeon and the operating room staff compared with traditional fluoroscopy.[39–41] Some pediatric studies suggest that the use of intraoperative CT should be used where the benefit is the greatest.[41] Nevertheless, because of the lower radiation sensitivity of the tissues exposed, the increased radiation exposure might not be a limiting factor of clinical relevance in the use of CT-CAOS on the equine foot.

In recent years, there have been advances in the CT technology used in equids, especially in overcoming the challenges of undertaking CT scans on the standing horse. These systems use either fan-beam technology or cone-beam technology (CBCT). The former is the standard technology used in clinical CT scanners and acquires volumetric image information; the latter is able to image larger body areas faster but does not generally make a full rotation around the patient. The Equina (Asto CT, Madison, Wisconsin) CT scanner uses fan-beam technology and allows imaging the head and the distal limbs on the standing sedated patient (**Fig. 7**).[42] The standing equine CT system used at the University of Pennsylvania in partnership with 4DDI Equine (Equimagine *TM*, Holbrook, New York) and currently maintained by Orimtech (Buffalo Grove, Illinois), uses a CBCT system coupled to robotic arms that rotates up to 190° around the region of interest as the images are being acquired (**Fig. 8**). In addition, this system offers digital radiography, fluoroscopy, and tomosynthesis image acquisition modes. Despite this advance in technology, its applications still are developing and currently imaging of the distal limbs up to the carpus and tarsus,

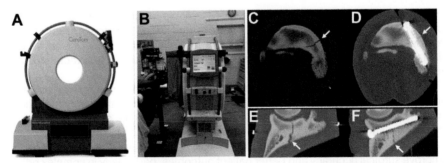

Fig. 5. (*A*) CereTom 8-slice small-bore mobile CT scanner from NeuroLogica-Samsung (14 Electronics Ave., Danvers, MA 01923, USA), with permission. (*B*) Intraoperative setting with the CereTom CT scanner for a distal phalanx fracture on an anesthetized horse. Intraoperative transverse (*C*) and sagittal (*E*) images in bone algorithm centered on the distal phalanx with an articular fracture (*arrows*). (*I*) intraoperative transverse (*D*) and sagittal (*F*) images in bone algorithm centered on the distal phalanx with reduction of the fracture seen on (*C*) and (*E*) (*arrows*). (*Courtesy of* Dr. Kyla Ortved and Dr. Kate Wulster from New Bolton Center University of Pennsylvania.)

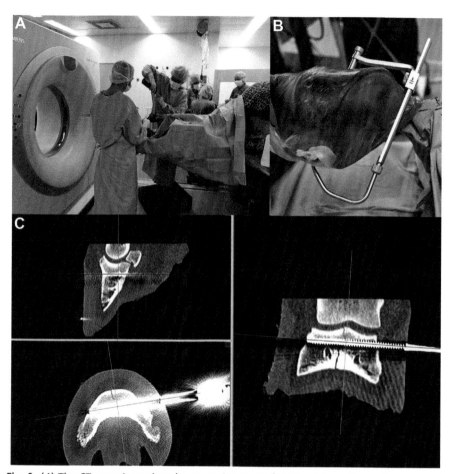

Fig. 6. (*A*) The CT room is used as the operation room for CT-guided orthopedic surgery at the equine clinic of the University of Zurich. In this system, the horse lies on a fixed CT table and the CT gantry moves back and forth around the foot to acquire the images as needed during the procedure. (*B*) Close look at the aiming device used for increased precision fixation of a pedal fracture in a horse. (*C*) Intraoperative display of the CT images in the sagittal (*top left*), transverse (*bottom left*), and dorsal (*right*) planes improves the visualization of the fracture and the quality of the fracture reduction and fixation. (*Courtesy of* Dr Michelle Jackson from the University of Zurich.)

the head, and the full neck can be acquired. More detailed information on these systems is provided by Wulster.[43]

CT is the gold standard for imaging bony structures and mineralization, but MRI is better for imaging the soft tissue structures. The contrast of the soft tissues on CT scans, however, greatly improves with the use of positive contrast media. Nonselective CT angiography is the standard imaging technique for vascular assessment in trauma patients and has been used successfully in horses with trauma to the distal limb to assess the arterial flow.[44] In these horses, 578 mg Iodine/kg to 658 mg Iodine/kg were administered via 1 or 2 jugular vein catheters. Because of the large size of the equine patient, the regional administration of positive contrast media can reduce the overall contrast dose to the patient and the cost of the study as well as

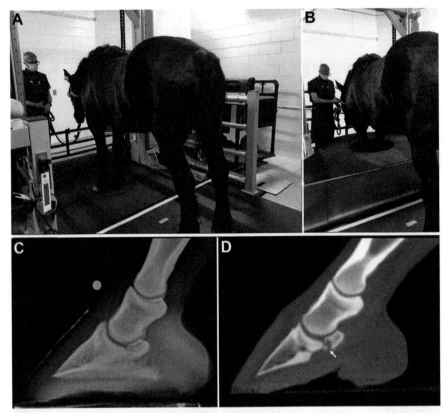

Fig. 7. (A) A sedated horse stands on the Asto CT Equina scanner's platform, ready for image acquisition. (B) During image acquisition, the gantry displaces proximally as images of the distal limb are acquired. (C) Lateromedial radiographs of the foot on a 11-year-old Lipizzaner with no obvious abnormality. (D) Sagittal CT images in bone algorithm on the same horse as (C), depicting fragmentation of the distal border of the navicular bone (arrow). (Courtesy of Dr. Sabrina H. Brounts from the University of Wisconsin-Madison.)

increase the contrast distribution in the anatomic region of interest. Administration of iodinated contrast medium at the medial palmar artery at the level of the carpus and improved the evaluation of the DDFT and the collateral ligaments of the distal interphalangeal joint as well as the distal interphalangeal synovium, the distal sesamoidean impar ligament, and the collateral sesamoidean ligament.[45–47] In addition, contrast-enhanced CT can identify more lesions in the foot than low-field MRI, with most lesions localized to the DDFT, and performs better than noncontrast CT identifying lesions at the DDFT insertion, with an overall sensitivity for detecting DDFT lesions of 93%.[47,48] CT is likely to miss bone edema and lesions, however, distal to the navicular bone.[46] Additional contrast techniques include the administration of contrast within synovial spaces, such as the distal interphalangeal joint,[49] the navicular bursa,[49] and the DDFT sheath,[50] which improves the visualization of the mesotendons and the plantar annular ligaments compared with noncontrast CT or radiography. Positively charged iodinated contrast media are being developed with the hope that these will penetrate the negatively charged glycosaminoglycan of the hyaline cartilage better than the current contrast media, and allow a quantitative assessment of the articular cartilage injury.[51]

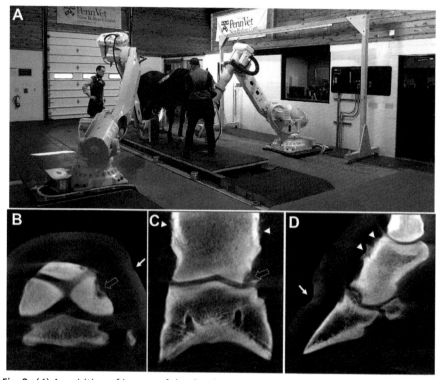

Fig. 8. (*A*) Acquisition of images of the distal aspect of the limb in a standing sedated horse with the robotic CBCT system at New Bolton Center, University of Pennsylvania. CT images of the distal aspect of the limb in bone algorithm in transverse (*B*), dorsal (*C*), and sagittal (*D*) planes, in a horse with a penetrating articular trauma and a secondary distolateral articular osteolytic lesion centered on the second phalanx (*black arrows*) and extensive periosteal reaction (*arrowheads*). Notice the defect at the dorsolateral margin of the hoof (*white arrows*). (*Courtesy of* Dr. Kyla Ortved and Dr. Kate Wulster from New Bolton Center University of Pennsylvania.)

Standing CT systems allow an increase in the accuracy of the diagnostics and the management of horses with foot pain, including those with laminitis, in which the status of the horny layer and the bone can be assessed better.[52] In addition, the performance of 3-D CT venogram studies on the standing horse will allow better visualization of the vascular anatomic disturbances within the foot and improved understanding of the pathophysiology of this disease.

MAGNETIC RESONANCE IMAGING

MRI is the gold standard for imaging soft tissues and bone edema and is of greatest value managing pathologic conditions of the foot.[53] In equine practice, standing MRI minimizes the risks and costs of general anesthesia at the expense of using low-strength magnetic fields. This also results in longer studies, lower image quality, and limited sequences. The use of high-strength magnetic field MRI leads to higher image resolution, faster scanning, and advanced imaging sequences but requires the equine patient to be under general anesthesia.[54]

Increased signal on short tau inversion recovery sequence (STIR) frequently is observed at the dorsal aspect of the distal phalanx; and, although it can be present both in lame and sound horses, larger areas of hyperintensity tend to be present in lame horses.[55] Besides, STIR signal at the insertion of the DDFT did not appear to influence the prognosis in 26 cases.[56]

MRI allows a more extensive assessment of the quality of the joint cartilage than with arthroscopy alone. Unfortunately, this can be achieved only with high-field magnets and special sequences, such as delayed gadolinium-enhanced MRI of cartilage (dGEMRIC) or T2-weighted mapping.[51,53,57,58] The former can accurately detect the glycosaminoglycan concentration of hyaline cartilage and, therefore, it is thought to be able to detect the early stages of osteoarthritis. In a recent study, dGEMRIC was able to differentiate varying degrees of naturally occurring osteoarthrosis in the distal interphalangeal joint.[59] In humans, more advanced sequences, such as sodium imaging, are used in the assessment of joint cartilage. The application of these sequences in equine diagnostic imaging is expected as the availability of higher-field MRI magnets ($\geq$3T) increases.[51]

The use of magic angle imaging can be used in conventional MRI systems to create T1 maps of the distal DDFT, with increased T1 values associated with increased sulfated glycosaminoglycan content and, therefore, with degenerative changes in the tendon matrix.[60]

A high proportion of lesions in the collateral ligaments of the distal interphalangeal joint are located distal to the coronary band.[61] The use of MRI-guided injection of these ligaments was superior to radiographic guidance in a cadaveric study and was completed safely in horses standing in a low-field magnet.[62] The use of MRI guidance for injection of PRPs at an insertional lesion of the DDFT has also been described recently in an anesthetized horse as a safe and likely more accurate technique compared with CT or ultrasound guidance, allowing diagnosis and treatment during the same anesthetic procedure.[63]

Standing MRI also has the potential to aid in the early diagnosis and management of laminitis. As opposed to CT, a 0.4T MRI was able to depict inflammation of the laminar corium and tendon edema as well as the loss of the dorsal aspect of the cortical bone of the distal phalanx and sclerosis.[52] Earlier studies highlighted the value of high-field MRI visualizing the laminae and identifying signal intensity and architectural changes within the corium and laminae, with strong association with the histologic diagnosis of active laminitis. In addition, the measurements obtained with magnetic resonance were more sensitive and specific predictors of laminitis than those obtained radiographically, and MRI was able to depict more lesions than radiographs alone.

Orthopedic MRI studies normally are performed without administration of contrast medium. Recent studies suggest, however, that there might be a benefit to its use, particularly for the identification of lesions in the foot. The administration of gadolinium to the palmar/plantar digital veins, as part of regional limb perfusion MRI, increased the detection of lesions in the foot, especially the collateral sesamoidean and impar ligaments, and the identification of neovascularization of the DDFT.[64] Neovascularization was most notable in horses with penetrating street nail injuries and was noted proximally at the level of the collateral sesamoidean ligament even if the penetrating trauma was at the level of the tendinous insertion. Other investigators have concluded that for the detection of pathologies in the equine foot, regional intra-arterial administration of gadolinium via the radial artery is a better choice than combined intravenous and arterial administration or intravenous administration alone, given its higher ratio of contrast enhancement and the lower volumes of contrast agent required. A more intense enhancement was observed in both pathologic and nonpathologic regions; the normal regions with greater increase in signal postregional arterial administration of contrast were the DDFT, navicular spongiosa, and peritendinous tissues.[65]

FUTURE ADVANCES IN DIAGNOSTIC IMAGING

The evolution of technology has led to the development of new diagnostic imaging tools and the advancement of older modalities like radiology. The greatest advancements will focus on data analysis and artificial intelligence (AI). The use of complex mathematical algorithms and deep learning has applications in veterinary diagnostic imaging, with a focus on the interpretation of small animal thoracic radiographs.[66,67] AI technology will help the radiologists improve their diagnostic accuracy, screening imaging studies with findings that require additional attention, and prevent errors and observer fatigue. AI will have a major role in identifying novel and patient specific therapies as well as predicting the clinical outcome of patients based on a combined analysis of clinical data sets, genomics, and medical images, such as radiographs, CT, and MRI, and also histopathology. The development and use of AI are limited by the large amount of data sets needed, the elevated cost of its development, and the absence of long-term follow-up studies, as examples. Consequently, these limitations should warrant caution on the use of the AI tools by veterinarians, particularly with steps in the early clinical uses of this technology.

CLINICS CARE POINTS

- The use of optimized radiographic projections can reduce the radiation exposure of the veterinarians and technicians while maintaining the diagnostic quality of the studies.
- Standing CT and PET scanners are meant to revolutionize the diagnosis and management of equine foot diseases.
- High-field MRI and contrast MRI are superior to low-field MRI in the diagnosis of pathology of the cartilage, ligaments, and hoof lamina.

DISCLOSURE

The author has nothing to disclose.

REFERENCES

1. Staples E. Evaluating the effect of two different points of X-ray beam centering on multiple radiographic measurements of the equine distal limb. Abstract presented at the: ACVR IVRA Joint Scientific Conference; October 14–19, 2018; Fort Worth, Texas.
2. Joostens Z, Evrad L, Olivier L, Busoni V. Effect of unipodal vs. bipodal stance on radiographic evaluation of forefeet in horses. Abstract presented at the: EVDI Annual Conference; August 31-September 3, 2016; Wroclaw, Poland.
3. Evrad L, Denoix JM, Rabba S, Busoni V. Evaluation of distal interphalangeal joint synovial effusion on radiographs: an ex vivo study on 12 equine feet. Abstract presented at the: EVDI Annual Conference; August 31-September 3, 2016; Wroclaw, Poland.
4. Whitlock J, Dixon J, Sherlock C, et al. Technical innovation changes standard radiographic protocols in veterinary medicine: is it necessary to obtain two dorsoproximal–palmarodistal oblique views of the equine foot when using computerised radiography systems? Vet Rec 2016;178(21):531.
5. Redden RF, Smith A. Understanding the Principles of Using Radiographs for Pathological Trimming and Shoeing. Proceedings 66th Annual Convention of the American Association of Equine Practitioners; December 1-18, 2020; Virtual..

6. Dyson S. Radiological interpretation of the navicular bone: Radiological interpretation of the navicular bone. Equine Vet Educ 2011;23(2):73–87.

7. Redden RF. Radiographic imaging of the equine foot. Vet Clin North Am Equine Pract 2003;19(2):379–92.

8. Hinkle FE, Johnson SA, Selberg KT, et al. A review of normal radiographical variants commonly mistaken for pathological findings in horses. Equine Vet Educ 2019. https://doi.org/10.1111/eve.13088. eve.13088.

9. Berry CR, Pool RR, Stover S, et al. Radiographic/morphologic investigation of a radiolucent crescent within the flexor central eminence of the navicular bone in thoroughbreds. Am J Vet Res 1992;53(9):1604–11.

10. Wright IM. A study of 118 cases of navicular disease: radiological features. Equine Vet J 1993;25(6):493–500.

11. Johnson SA, Barrett MF, Frisbie DD. Additional palmaroproximal-palmarodistal oblique radiographic projections improve accuracy of detection and characterization of equine flexor cortical lysis. Vet Radiol Ultrasound 2018;59(4):387–95.

12. Tivey M-EL, Van Dijk J, Dyson S. Extensive ossification of the ungular cartilages and other osseous abnormalities of the proximal and distal phalanges. Equine Vet Educ 2020;32(S10):25–30.

13. Clements PE, Handel I, McKane SA, et al. An investigation into the association between plantar distal phalanx angle and hindlimb lameness in a UK population of horses. Equine Vet Educ 2020;32(S10):52–9.

14. Pezzanite L, Bass L, Kawcak C, et al. The relationship between sagittal hoof conformation and hindlimb lameness in the horse. Equine Vet J 2019;51(4): 464–9.

15. Rowan C. The effect of radioopaque markers to delineate the dorsal hoof wall on image quality in digital equine radiograph. Abstract presented at the: EVDI Annual Conference; August 31-September 3, 2016; Wroclaw, Poland.

16. Mullard J, Ireland J, Dyson S. Radiographic assessment of the ratio of the hoof wall distal phalanx distance to palmar length of the distal phalanx in 415 front feet of 279 horses. Equine Vet Educ 2020;32(S10):2–10.

17. Kramer J, Rucker A, Leise B. Venographic evaluation of the circumflex vessels and lamellar circumflex junction in laminitic horses. Equine Vet Educ 2020; 32(7):386–92.

18. Trolinger-Meadows KD, Morton AJ, McCarrel TM. Digital Venography Including the 60o- Dorsoproximopalmarodistal Oblique Radiographic Projection to Evaluate Non-Laminitic Foot Disease in Horses. Abstract presented at the: ACVS Surgery Summit; October 24-27, 2018; Phoenix, AZ.

19. Shields GE. Comparison of ultrasound vs. magnetic resonance imaging for detection of soft tissue injuries in the palmar aspect of the equine foot. Abstract presented at the: ACVR Annual Scientific Conference; October 18-21, 2017; Phoenix, AZ.

20. Maleas G, Mageed M, Gerlach K. Comparison of ultrasound, bursography, MRI, and bursoscopy as diagnostic tools for navicular apparatus pathology in nine horses. Abstract presented at the: EVDI Congress; August 21-24, 2019; Basel, Switzerland.

21. Evaluation of Nuclear Scintigraphy As A Diagnostic Test In Lame And Poorly Performing Sports Horses. Equine Vet J 2017;49:19.

22. Fischer DR. Musculoskeletal Imaging Using Fluoride PET. Semin Nucl Med 2013; 43(6):427–33.

23. Even-Sapir E, Mishani E, Flusser G, et al. 18F-Fluoride Positron Emission Tomography and Positron Emission Tomography/Computed Tomography. Semin Nucl Med 2007;37(6):462–9.

24. Spriet M. Validation of a Dedicated standing equine PET scanner and early data in 61 racehorses. Abstract presented at the: ACVR Annual Scientific Conference; October 19-23, 2020; Virtual.

25. Ortved K. Advances in the Clinical Applications of Equine Imaging. Conference session presented at the: ACVR Annual Scientific Conference; October 19-23, 2020; Virtual.

26. Spriet M, Espinosa P, Kyme AZ, et al. 18F-sodium fluoride positron emission tomography of the equine distal limb: Exploratory study in three horses. Equine Vet J 2018;50(1):125–32.

27. Wilson S. Evaluation of 18F-FDG positron emission tomography for assessment of the deep digital flexor tendon in the equine foot. Abstract presented at the: ACVR Annual Scientific Conference; October 19-23, 2020; Virtual.

28. Spriet M, Espinosa-Mur P, Cissell DD, et al. 18F-sodium fluoride positron emission tomography of the racing Thoroughbred fetlock: Validation and comparison with other imaging modalities in nine horses. Equine Vet J 2019;51(3):375–83.

29. Spriet M. Enthesopathy of the chondrosesamoidean ligament on the distal phalanx in horses: Retrospective study of 20 positron emission tomography cases. Abstract presented at the: ACVR Annual Scientific Conference; October 18-21, 2017; Phoenix, AZ.

30. Sannajust K. Normal Standardized Uptake Values and Attenuation Correction for 18F-Sodium Fluoride PET of the Equine Distal Limb. Abstract presented at the: ACVR Annual Scientific Conference; October 19-23, 2020; Virtual.

31. Spriet M. 18F-FDG PET for assessment of the hoof lamina in normal, laminitic, and lame horses. Abstract presented at the: EVDI Congress; August 31-September 3, 2019; Basel, Switzerland.

32. Claerhoudt S, Bergman EHJ, Saunders JH. Computed Tomographic Anatomy of the Equine Foot. Anat Histol Embryol 2014;43(5):395–402.

33. Preux M, Klopfenstein Bregger MD, Brünisholz HP, et al. Clinical use of computer-assisted orthopedic surgery in horses. Vet Surg 2020;49(6):1075–87.

34. Katzman SA, Spriet M, Galuppo LD. Outcome following computed tomographic imaging and subsequent surgical removal of keratomas in equids: 32 cases (2005-2016). J Am Vet Med Assoc 2019;254(2):266–74.

35. Milner PI. Decision making with keratomas: How advanced imaging can advance your cause. Equine Vet Educ 2020;32(6):311–2.

36. Waschke A, Walter J, Duenisch P, et al. CT-navigation versus fluoroscopy-guided placement of pedicle screws at the thoracolumbar spine: single center experience of 4,500 screws. Eur Spine J 2013;22(3):654–60.

37. Heer C, Fürst AE, Del Chicca F, et al. Comparison of 3D-assisted surgery and conservative methods for treatment of type III fractures of the distal phalanx in horses. Equine Vet Educ 2020;32(S10):42–51.

38. Jackson MA, Fürst AE. The use of an aiming device and computed tomography for treatment of articular pedal bone fractures in horses. Abstract presented at the: ECVS 28th Annual Scientific Meeting; July 4-6, 2019; Budapest, Hungary.

39. Riis J, Lehman RR, Perera RA, et al. A retrospective comparison of intraoperative CT and fluoroscopy evaluating radiation exposure in posterior spinal fusions for scoliosis. Patient Saf Surg 2017;11:32.

40. Mendelsohn D, Strelzow J, Dea N, et al. Patient and surgeon radiation exposure during spinal instrumentation using intraoperative computed tomography-based navigation. Spine J 2016;16(3):343–54.

41. Dabaghi Richerand A, Christodoulou E, Li Y, et al. Comparison of Effective Dose of Radiation During Pedicle Screw Placement Using Intraoperative Computed Tomography Navigation Versus Fluoroscopy in Children With Spinal Deformities. J Pediatr Orthop 2016;36(5):530–3.

42. Brounts S. Imaging of distal limbs of the sedated standing horse using a novel vertical robotic helical fan beam computed tomography system. Abstract presented at the: Annual Scientific Meeting of the ECVS; July 2, 2020; Virtual.

43. Wulster KB. Diagnosis of Skeletal Injury in the Sport Horse. Vet Clin North Am Equine Pract 2018;34(2):193–213.

44. Walker WT, Ducharme NG, Tran J, et al. Nonselective computed tomography angiography for detecting arterial blood flow to the distal limb following trauma in two small equids. Equine Vet Educ 2017;29(1):15–21.

45. Puchalski SM, Galuppo LD, Hornof WJ, et al. Intraarterial contrast-enhanced computed tomography of the equine distal extremity. Vet Radiol Ultrasound 2007;48(1):21–9.

46. Vallance SA, Bell RJW, Spriet M, et al. Comparisons of computed tomography, contrast enhanced computed tomography and standing low-field magnetic resonance imaging in horses with lameness localised to the foot. Part 1: anatomic visualisation scores. Equine Vet J 2012;44(1):51–6.

47. Vallance SA, Bell RJW, Spriet M, et al. Comparisons of computed tomography, contrast-enhanced computed tomography and standing low-field magnetic resonance imaging in horses with lameness localised to the foot. Part 2: Lesion identification. Equine Vet J 2012;44(2):149–56.

48. van Hamel SE, Bergman HJ, Puchalski SM, et al. Contrast-enhanced computed tomographic evaluation of the deep digital flexor tendon in the equine foot compared to macroscopic and histological findings in 23 limbs. Equine Vet J 2014;46(3):300–5.

49. Pauwels F, Hartmann A, al-Alawneh J. Diagnostic utility of 105 distal extremity contrast enhanced computed tomographic examinations in the horse. Abstract presented at the: EVDI Congress; August 21-24, 2019; Basel, Switzerland.

50. Computed Tomographic Contrast Tenography Of The Digital Flexor Tendon Sheath Of The Equine Hindlimb: Improving Preoperative Diagnostic Techniques. Equine Vet J 2017;49:17.

51. Nelson BB, Kawcak CE, Barrett MF, et al. Recent advances in articular cartilage evaluation using computed tomography and magnetic resonance imaging. Equine Vet J 2018;50(5):564–79. https://doi.org/10.1111/evj.12808.

52. YAMADA K, INUI T, ITOH M, et al. Characteristic findings of magnetic resonance imaging (MRI) and computed tomography (CT) for severe chronic laminitis in a Thoroughbred horse. J Equine Sci 2017;28(3):105–10.

53. Barrett MF, Frisbie DD, King MR, et al. A review of how magnetic resonance imaging can aid in case management of common pathological conditions of the equine foot. Equine Vet Educ 2017;29(12):683–93.

54. Morgan JM. Morbidity Associated with Equine MRI Under General Anesthesia. Abstract presented at the: ACVS Surgery Summit; October 16-19, 2019; Las Vegas, NV.

55. Vandersmissen M, Evrard L, Busoni V. Prevalence and distribution of distal phalanx short-tau inversion recovery hypersignal on magnetic resonance images of

129 equine feet. Abstract presented at the: EVDI Congress; August 21-24, 2019; Basel, Switzerland.

56. Taylor S. Imaging findings and clinical follow up of horses with insertional deep digital flexor tendinopathy with or without associated enthesiopathy. Abstract presented at the: EVDI Congress; August 21-24, 2019; Basel, Switzerland.

57. Rovel T, Audigié F, Coudry V, et al. Evaluation of standing low-field magnetic resonance imaging for diagnosis of advanced distal interphalangeal primary degenerative joint disease in horses: 12 cases (2010–2014). J Am Vet Med Assoc 2019; 254(2):257–65.

58. Cissell DD. Regional variation in quantitative magnetic resonance imaging of equine distal interphalangeal joint cartilage. Abstract presented at the: ACVR Annual Scientific Conference; October 2017; Phoenix, AZ.

59. Bischofberger AS, Fürst AE, Torgerson PR, et al. Use of a 3-Telsa magnet to perform delayed gadolinium-enhanced magnetic resonance imaging of the distal interphalangeal joint of horses with and without naturally occurring osteoarthritis. Am J Vet Res 2018;79(3):287–98.

60. Spriet M. Magnetic resonance t1-mapping of the equine distal deep digital flexor tendon. Abstract presented at the: EVDI Annual Conference; August 31-September 3, 2016; Wroclaw, Poland.

61. Beasley B, Selberg K, Giguère S, et al. Magnetic resonance imaging characterisation of lesions within the collateral ligaments of the distal interphalangeal joint – 28 cases. Equine Vet Educ 2020;32(S10):11–7.

62. White NA, Barrett JG. Magnetic Resonance Imaging-Guided Treatment of Equine Distal Interphalangeal Joint Collateral Ligaments: 2009–2014. Front Vet Sci 2016; 3. https://doi.org/10.3389/fvets.2016.00073.

63. Marcatili M, Marshall J, Voute L. Magnetic resonance imaging-guided injection of platelet-rich plasma for treatment of an insertional core lesion of the deep digital flexor tendon within the foot of a horse. Equine Vet Educ 2018;30(8):409–14.

64. Aarsvold S, Solano M, Garcia-Lopez J. Magnetic resonance imaging following regional limb perfusion of gadolinium contrast medium in 26 horses. Equine Vet J 2018;50(5):649–57.

65. Zani DD, Rabbogliatti V, Ravasio G, et al. Contrast enhanced magnetic resonance imaging of the foot in horses using intravenous versus regional intraarterial injection of gadolinium. Open Vet J 2018;8(4):471–8.

66. Boissady E, Comble A de L, Zhu X, et al. Artificial intelligence evaluating primary thoracic lesions has an overall lower error rate compared to veterinarians or veterinarians in conjunction with the artificial intelligence. Vet Radiol Ultrasound 2020;61(6):619–27.

67. Li S, Wang Z, Visser LC, et al. Pilot study: Application of artificial intelligence for detecting left atrial enlargement on canine thoracic radiographs. Vet Radiol Ultrasound 2020;61(6):611–8.

Mechanical Principles of the Equine Foot

Raul Bras, DVM, CJF, Scott Morrison, DVM*

KEYWORDS

- Foot • Gait analysis • Laminitis • Mechanics • Radiography • Shoeing techniques
- Venogram

KEY POINTS

- Techniques for evaluating foot mechanics and balance in real time
- Shoeing techniques to support the injured/diseased foot
- Prophylactic shoeing techniques—minimizing stress on the foot in high-level competition horses

EVALUATING EQUINE FOOT MECHANICS

For a foot to remain healthy and accommodate its basic functions, it requires proper form and structure. *Balance* is the term used when describing a foot's form and structure. A balanced foot is functionally efficient and capable of accommodating the basic purposes of the foot; support, shock, absorption, traction and proprioception. Balance can be categorized further as dynamic and static. Static balance of the foot evaluates its geometric shape and the orientation of the internal and external structures and evaluated in 3 different planes: frontal, sagittal, and transverse. Dynamic balance assesses the flight and stance phases when a horse is in motion.

Throughout history, the concepts of balance have been taught and applied as they are understood and largely dependent on visual inspection of the horse's conformation, gait, and hoof geometry. Centerlines, proportions, and trimming to the limb axis are some of the basic principles of balance that guide hoof trimming/shoeing. The simplicity of traditional techniques cannot diminish the importance and reliability of these fundamental principles.

Today, additional technologies are available to evaluate foot balance and include radiology, pressure sensors, videography, accelerometers, and gyroscopes, force plates and slow-motion videography. Several of these technologies, however, are research tools and not easily available to the practitioner.

Equine Podiatry, Rood & Riddle Equine Hospital, PO Box 12070, Lexington, KY 40580, USA
* Corresponding author.
E-mail address: smorrison@roodandriddle.com

Vet Clin Equine 37 (2021) 581–618
https://doi.org/10.1016/j.cveq.2021.09.001
0749-0739/21/© 2021 Elsevier Inc. All rights reserved.

Static Balance

Evaluating the foot statically is the method of evaluation used most often and provides the practitioner insight into how the foot is loaded and behaves dynamically. A balanced foot is not perfectly symmetric, simply because the forces loading the foot are not symmetric, however, the foot should have a degree of symmetry and be distortion-free, for example, flares, dishes, bull-nosed dorsal wall, crushed/collapsed wall, contracted heel, and displaced coronary band. Any foot distortion is a sign of imbalance and are the result of either overloading or underloading an area of the hoof and indicates structural failure of a section of the hoof capsule. A distorted hoof does not respond well to normal loading forces and is susceptible to trauma and injury.[1–6] Therefore, the importance of foot shape and balance is vital to maintaining soundness and optimal performance.

Hoof shape is related directly to the position of the pedal bone and how internal structures are loaded and interact with the ground. The distal interphalangeal joint (DIP) is the major joint of the digit and the center of articulation about which many structures of the distal limb impact during movement. The DIP joint, therefore, is considered a focal point of the digit and a major landmark when assessing hoof form, function, and balance. The DIP is affected adversely by asymmetric loading patterns when moving on uneven ground and also is influenced by foot treatments, such as trimming and shoeing. The position of the pedal bone and the way it articulates with the DIP joint in 3 planes, directly affects the flexor and extensor moment arms of the digital flexor and extensor tendons, medial/lateral joint space, and stress and strain on the supporting structures of the digit. Pedal bone orientation and DIP joint articulation are integral parts of foot balance evaluation and radiology have been shown useful tools in evaluating foot balance.

Radiography

Radiographic evaluation of the equine foot is useful to evaluate static balance because it clearly demonstrates the position of the bones and the hoof capsule and their relationship to the ground surface. Routine parameters measured on a radiographic image are sole depth, phalangeal alignment, palmer/plantar angle, horn-lamellar zone (HLZ)/dorsal hoof wall thickness, bone angle, coronary band to extensor process distance (CED), angle of flexor surface of navicular bone, center of rotation, center of articulation, joint spacing, dorsal hoof wall hoof angle, and heel angle. Diagnostic radiographs require proper technique with the horse standing square and balanced on all 4 limbs, with the head and neck positioned facing forward. Both feet should be on blocks in a normal position replicating the horse's natural stance. Turning the horse's head, unilateral weight bearing, and adduction and abduction of the limb when performing radiographs all affect DIP joint articulation and joint space.[7,8]

Some properties of foot balance vary with limb conformation and are subjective; however, the balanced foot possess the following characteristics.

- Even joint space on dorsopalmer/plantar standing radiograph of the DIP joint
- Straight hoof pastern axis—studies using instrumented horseshoes and moving on a treadmill at a walk, trot, and canter revealed that forces at the toe, medial heel, and lateral heel were the lowest when the hoof and pastern regions were aligned.[9]
- Center of rotation of the DIP joint or widest part of foot should be in the center of the weight-bearing surface of the shoe in the sagittal plane.
- Palmer angle of pedal bone should be between 2° and 5°.

- Heel position should be located at the widest part of the frog.
- Heel angle should be within 5° of toe angle.
- Solar surface of foot perpendicular to long axis of pastern bone
- Even hoof wall growth from all parts of the coronary band

A preventative hoof care program should be implemented to manage and respond to signs of hoof capsule distortion effectively before they cause lameness. Shoeing strategies to manage unbalanced feet are discussed later.

Dynamic Balance

The point of ground contact affects the way the foot and all the structures proximal are loaded with symmetry and cadence, the characteristics desired in equine athletes. These are the essential concepts underlying the importance of dynamic balance. Cases should be evaluated at the walk and trot before and after trimming/shoeing.

In general, horses land heel first, particularly at higher speeds, and use the shock-absorbing function of the heel. At the walk, landing flat or heel first is considered normal, whereas toe-first landing is considered abnormal and increases peak strain on the deep digital flexor tendon (DDFT) and navicular bone.[10] Following ground impact, the foot slides slightly and comes to a stop as the body passes over the limb in midstance. In a limb with good conformation, the foot should land directly beneath the boney column when traveling in a straight line. This provides stability and support during midstance.

During stance phase, the trajectory of the center of pressure (COP) travels from the heel toward the toe. As the stored energy in the fetlock's suspensory apparatus is released, after midstance, the limb springs forward and upward and the heels begin to lift off, initiating breakover or heel lift. The breakover phase begins with heel lift and ends when the toe leaves the ground. As the foot leaves the ground, it enters the flight phase of the stride. The trajectory of the flight pattern of the foot is a biphasic (double-humped) parabolic curve despite the often-portrayed rendition of hoof flight as a uniphasic (single-humped) parabolic curve.[9,11]

Signs of dynamic imbalance are obvious asymmetries in any phase of the gait, limb interference, toe-first landing, and obvious medial or lateral landing, twisting, or bowing of the limb when traveling in a straight line. Lameness creates a dynamic imbalance either as a cause or a result and should be taken into consideration during the evaluation.

TECHNIQUES FOR ASSESSING FOOT MECHANICS IN REAL TIME

Technological advancements have been made to aid in the objective assessment of the horse in motion.[12] Force plates, pressure sensors, gyroscopes, accelerometers, and videography all are technologies to assist in the evaluation of the kinematics and dynamics of the horse's gait.

Force Plates or Platforms

Force plates/platforms directly measure force or ground reaction force. Force plates most commonly measure vertical force but some are capable of measuring force in multiple planes (X,Y,Z). Force plates typically are not large enough to capture multiple foot strikes of a horse and typically cannot describe the location of peak force/pressure under the hoof. Large force plates typically are available only at research institutions and not available to the practitioner.

Pressure Plates and Wireless Pressure Mapping Systems

Pressure mapping systems are commercially available to measure multiple points of contact simultaneously in a dynamic, detailed pressure map (**Fig. 1**) They provide a distribution of contact area, peak pressure data, relative force distribution, COP, and changes over time or over a gait cycle; the information is unattainable from force platforms. Pressure plates can measure force but only vertical force through the summation of all the sensors bearing weight and lead to less accuracy than force plates in measuring force.[13] Pressure mats are available to walk or trot over; however, these mats are designed for humans and are short in length, and it is difficult and impractical to use these commercial mats for equine gait analysis. The equine patient can stand on the pressure mats for static pressure mapping; however, the way in the horse is placed or positioned on the mat affects the pressure mapping pattern. It is more accurate to use a wireless in-shoe pressure mapping sensor, allowing the horse to move naturally, and likely leads to more accurate assessment. Wireless systems are available, which can read the sensors from 100 m away and scanning speeds up to 100 Hz (100 times/s). The sensor is a thin film placed between the sole surface of the hoof and the shoe, like a pad.[14] Horses can be walked, jogged in-hand, and ridden under tack and in different types of footings.

Inertial Sensors (Gyroscopes and Accelerometers)

A gyroscope measures the orientation and the rate of change in the position of the object it is mounted on, whereas accelerometers are devices used to measure forces of acceleration or change in velocity. Gyroscopes and accelerometers often are used together to analyze the position and speed of an object. There are wireless motion tracking systems available that can be mounted to the hoof. Data can be collected at 1140 Hz and transmitted to a laptop in real time.[15] Landing, breakover, stance, swing, timing, and relative hoof position can be tracked for each foot, and, in this way, symmetry between feet and comparisons before and after trimming/shoeing can be assessed.

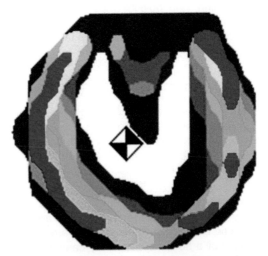

Fig. 1. Pressure plates provide a distribution of contact area, peak pressure data, relative force distribution, COP, and changes over time or over a gait cycle.

Video Gait Analysis

Videography is widely available and can help assess the movements of a horse. Ranging from expensive high-speed cameras to a simple smartphone, videography has become commonplace and easily available. It is helpful to slow down the video speed to analyze the characteristics of the gait. Slow-motion videography improves temporal resolution, particularly for hoof landing patterns. Software programs are available using motion tracking software with markers placed on anatomic parts of the horse. The software provides objective measurements as it tracks the markers. Joint angle, stride length, and hoof flight information are used comparatively in follow-up examinations after trimming/shoeing changes.

SHOEING TECHNIQUES TO SUPPORT THE INJURED/DISEASED FOOT
Laminitis

Equine podiatry is a professional field of service involving the dedicated efforts of responsible and knowledgeable foot-focused veterinarians and farriers serving the horse in both routine hoof care and supportive therapeutic plans when there is disease of the foot. Working with challenging cases, for example, laminitis can be rewarding and a unique experience when a good outcome is achieved. This involves a strong team commitment between farrier and veterinarian who are knowledgeable and skilled in equine podiatry.

Many teams struggle because of a lack of a 'knowledge' foundation in tested and evidence-based concepts and techniques and therefore with a correct clinical diagnosis and treatment plan. Fortunately, substantial progress has been made in equine podiatry bringing forward-thinking farriers and veterinarians together sharing information, collaboration, and similar goals for success. Many previous career-ending foot diseases today routinely are treated successfully, returning the horse to a healthy and comfortable life and athleticism.

This article focuses on proactive diagnostics and practical treatment methods for laminitis, emphasizing the principles of therapeutic shoeing based on foot mechanics by modifying the external and internal forces working on the laminitic foot to minimize developing pathology to the soft and hard foot tissues (**Fig. 2**). Recognizing the subtle changes early in the hoof capsule can indicate possible internal changes in the foot. A proactive approach commonly means the difference between success and failure in preserving the structural integrity of the foot.[16]

Therapeutic Shoeing: A Mechanical Thought Process

Therapeutic shoeing is used commonly as a prophylactic method for the prevention and treatment of various lamenesses, that is, laminitis[17,18] (**Fig. 3**). The primary goal for therapeutic application is to compensate for the presenting mechanical limitations of the distal limb and improve healing of the affected foot. The mechanical impact of trimming and shoeing for preventive and therapeutic purposes is poorly understood by many farriers and veterinarians. The importance in understanding the mechanical process(es) lies in the understanding of the internal and external forces acting on the foot, therefore, directly influencing the shape, strength, and resilience of the hoof capsule and reliability of the internal structures to survive and thrive. Thus, mechanical improvement can be used to alleviate excessive forces and increase digit support. Without understanding the mechanical forces in the foot that control the blood supply for horn growth, healing is compromised, and recurring problems continue in shoeing.

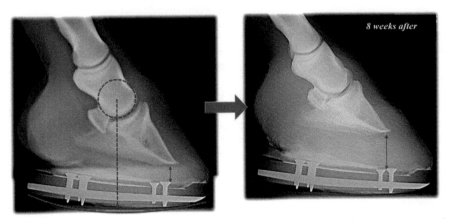

Fig. 2. Principles of therapeutic shoeing based on the mechanical thought process of altering the external and internal forces acting on the laminitic foot to mitigate developing pathology. Consideration of the forces within the foot influence the vital vascular supply, which ultimately enhance the healing environment. Circle shows Center of rotation. Bidirectional arrows shows Sole depth. Both left and right panels are of the 'right' foot.

The equine veterinarian's goal is the overall soundness of the horse, in parallel with the farrier focusing on health of the hoof capsule. A collaborative effort of each is needed for the best results when there are clinical foot problems. Veterinarians' and farriers' clinical expertise is achieved through years of experience, education, critical thinking, improved skills, team spirit, and strong work ethic.

Biomechanics of the Distal Limb and Farrier Science

A comprehensive understanding of farrier science and foot mechanics is helpful in making changes in foot support to enhance improvements in foot diseases, especially laminitis. The foot, protected by an external rigid integument—keratin—contains the suspensory apparatus, external caudal soft tissues, internal bony structure, tendon and ligament function, skin and integument, fibrocartilage, fascia, lamellar architecture, and vascular and nerve supply, with a complex set of mechanoreceptors.

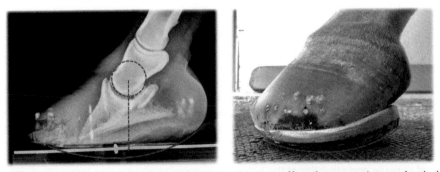

Fig. 3. The primary goal for therapeutic application is to offset the presenting mechanical limitations of the distal limb and enhance the healing environment. Hashed circle and vertical line shows Center of rotation. Concave line in both figures shows Goal of therapeutic showing to mechanically maximize center of rotation and maximize break over. Both images are the left foot.

This interconnected system of these structures permits the foot to function as a unified entity for locomotion and supporting the horse's body mass. It does this by dispersing the forces of ground impact and distributing load to prevent overuse and injury to any 1 component. In the healthy hoof, there is a robust blood supply to nurture laminae, bone, and soft tissues and to encourage normal hoof growth. Because of the interrelation of these digital structures, when 1 part is injured or permanently damaged due to genetic factors, overload, repetitive injury, disease, environmental factors, or human intervention, the whole foot is compromised. A cascade of events results in altered growth and hoof capsule distortion, because all parts are affected when 1 or more areas fail[19] (**Fig. 4**).

Mechanical Principles of the Laminitic Foot

To explain the value of applying biomechanical benefit to the laminitic foot, it can be considered as a method of changing load from load-induced vascular compromised tissue to healthier areas to stimulate healing in the affected areas. Digital radiography and venograms provide 2 excellent methods to maximize interpretive skills when managing a cascade of events in laminitis. The goal of these 2 techniques is to provide useful information for the veterinarian and farrier for treatment options. Principally, the goal is to relieve destructive forces that change foot mechanics and rob transport of nutrients to injured tissue. Positive tissue response and prognosis depend on the severity of the laminitis, before the start of treatment measures, and stopping the root cause of the disease.

Five important forces work on the digit: DDFT plays a major role (**Fig. 5**). Through its musculotendon unit, forces on the coffin bone are offset by opposing forces of robust laminae/bone/horn and, to a lesser extent, by the opposing forces exerted by the extensor tendon. This relationship of neutralizing forces between lamellar bonds and extensor versus flexor moments creates a sling situation for the coffin bone. This suspensory mechanism stabilizes and protects the digit under loading forces. The DDFT also contributes to the hemodynamics of blood circulation between limb loading cycles, all vital parts of the overall health and permanence of the foot.

In general, the goals of mechanical therapeutic shoeing and trimming are based on the relationship of the suspension and support components of the digit (**Fig. 6**). Oddly, reducing the tension of the DDFT relative to the severity of lamellar lesions and

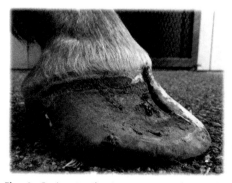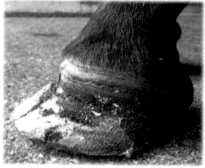

Fig. 4. Owing to the interconnectedness of the digital structures, when 1 component is weakened or permanently damaged, the entire hoof capsule is compromised, with a cascade of damage, altered growth, and hoof capsule distortions. Left figure is the 'Right foot' and the right figure is the 'Left foot'.

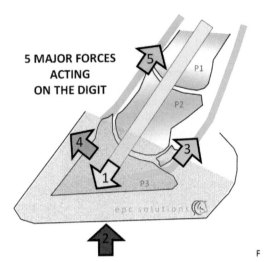

Fig. 5. Major forces in the equine foot are due to the downward load exerted by the weight of the horse through the bony column (yellow); proximal-palmar pull of the DDFT (green); pulling force of the common digital extensor tendon (purple); lamellar attachments between P3 and hoof wall (blue); and distal phalangeal supportive function by the sole and frog (red). (Courtesy of Sylvia Nemeth-Kornherr).

improving breakover to relieve influence caused by hoof distortion reduce forces generated around the center axis of foot. Reducing the tension of the DDFT lessens the shearing forces on the diseased lamellar in the weakened, laminitic foot and diminishes solar compression affecting the corium and blood vessels. Lessening DDFT tension is achieved by therapeutic trimming and shoeing techniques using the mechanical advantage via 4 areas: (1) reducing concussion to the foot by providing solar relief and support; (2) shifting load away from painful or compromised parts to

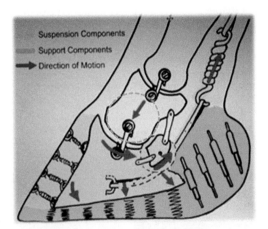

Fig. 6. In general, the goals of mechanical therapeutic shoeing and trimming are based on the relationship of the suspension and support components of the digit. Reducing the tension of the DDFT relative to the intensity of the lamellar lesions will minimize forces generated around the center axis of rotation of the foot. Meaning of colors are explained in the figure in the upper left hand corner. (Courtesy of Dr. Ric Redden).

healthier areas; (3) modifying the distribution of force; and (4) changing the smoothness of movement through the DIP.

Diagnostic Tools: Podiatry—Standard of Care—Radiographic Protocol

The art of podiatry has a fundamental learning curve that begins with an understanding of the internal and external parts of the foot that support form and function. The external hoof capsule is important in understanding the foot radiographs of the internal structures, completes the information needed for best foot care decisions, and an important aid for trimming and use of therapeutic shoes[20] (**Fig. 7**). The specific radiographic views permit measuring and assessing the soft and hard tissues of the digit without distortion, providing accurate measurements within a few degrees of angulation change in millimeters.6 The effects of changing hoof angles on distal limb joints has been described.[17,19,21]

The foot-specific radiographic protocols generate accurate, repeatable series of images for continuous monitoring throughout the course of the disease. These foot-specific radiographs differ from standard diagnostic views (**Fig. 8**) and include improved joint space definition. Calibrated, focal centered foot-specific radiographic protocols use a low-beam projection to areas of interest in the digit. Using the specific beam/horse/cassette orientation focuses on the area of interest with repeatable images and comparative views, offering a reliable means of identifying a large range of foot characteristics specifically tracked over time.

Foot radiographic images identify the interrelation of the distal limb: integrity of bone linking with horn, HLZ thickening, widening, or separating of the lamellar corium, white line disease, laminitic sequestrae and abscess tracking, laminar swelling, and distal descent of P3 with numerical measurements. The radiographic views include the following.

Podiatry-specific Images: Lateral-Medial View

The low-beam L-M (lateromedial) projection produces consistent, repeatable images of the soft tissue structures and includes sole depth and cup, palmar (plantar) angle

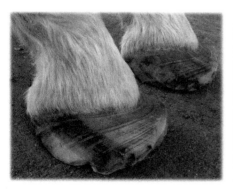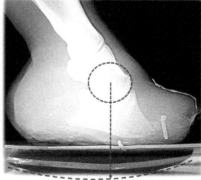

Fig. 7. A radiographic view into the internal structures completes the data required for optimal foot care decisions and selves as an important aid to trimming and application of therapeutic shoes. Circle, vertical line, and curved line represent the goal in support of the laminitic foot and the center of weigh-bearing. Left figure are the right foot (furthest away) and left foot (closest). Right image is the 'Right foot'.

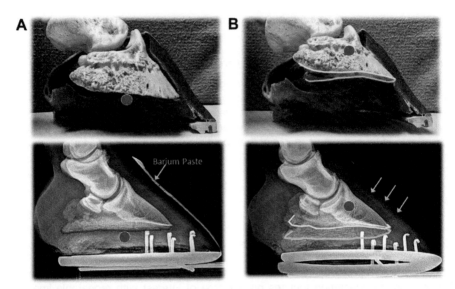

Fig. 8. Podiatry-specific radiographs. (*A*) Low beam produces superimposed wings, superimposed shoe branches and 1 block edge. This provides accurate linear and angle measurements. (*B*) Diagnostic view with focal beam aimed higher, often aimed at the navicular bone or toward the extensor process. Two coffin wings and 2 shoe branches are depicted. Block surface is oblique (edges and block face can be seen). Linear and angle measurements cannot be accurately assessed. Absent barium paste—x-ray bum out does not represent tine dorsal wall edge.Upper panel in A is a prosection with red dots depicting center of focal beam. Lower panel in A is the radiograph of prosection depicting the superimposition of lateral and medial edges of third phalanx used for angle measurements (red line). Upper panel in B is prosection with red dot (extensor process) and purple dot (navicular bone) and focal beam aimed higher to better assess lateral and medial edges of third phalanx (yellow and blue lines respectively). With the angulation accurate linear and angle measurements cannot be accurately made.

(PA), HLZ, Coronary band - extensor process distance (CED), and digital breakover (**Fig. 9**).

Podiatry-specific Images: Dorsopalmar (Anteroposterior) View

The DP/anteroposterior view is important to confirm quarter flaring, heel tubule bending (windswept), joint space impingement, and L-M (lateromedial) imbalances (**Fig. 10**).

The information obtained from foot radiographs, using the low-beam protocol, is of diagnostic and prognostic value, monitoring the efficacy and success of therapeutic trimming and shoeing programs. Veterinarians acquire collaboration with an experienced farrier in interpreting and executing a plan of treatment.

Measured parameters–objective data offer important information and include the PA, sole depth, and digital breakover for the farrier and provide guidance for mechanical realignment and limitations of the foot. As in the case of laminitis, there generally is a small margin for error and the difference between success and failure for the intended goal (**Fig. 11**).

The complex foot model can be divided into 2 components — suspension and support in building strong mechanics into the shoeing plan. The deep flexor muscle/tendon unit

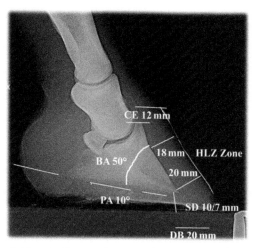

Fig. 9. The low-beam L-M projection produces consistent, comparable images of the soft tissue parameters, which hold valuable information for the veterinarian-farrier team. Podiatry radiograph are an excellent tool with quantitative measurements, therefore, a highly useful tool in assessing and monitoring any changes in the foot. BA, Bone angle; CE, coronary extensor process distance; DB, digital break over; HLZ, hoof-lamellar-zone; PA, palmar (plantar) angle; SD, sole depth.

is a key component of the suspension mechanism because of its attachment to the coffin bone is attached to the hoof capsule by the interdigitating laminae. Any compromise to laminae unfavorably affects the suspension mechanism; thus, mechanical use, to neutralize the forces of the DDFT, is needed.[22] The support component uses structures of the foot that complement the suspension component by behaving as an energy

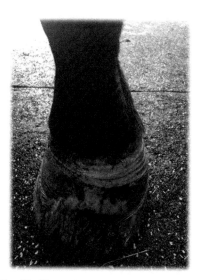
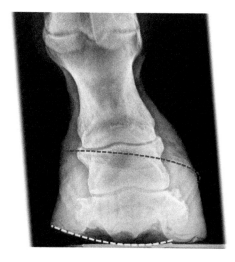

Fig. 10. The DP/anteroposterior view is an important adjunct to the lateral view to verify aspects, such as joint space impingement and mediolateral imbalances, especially in the laminitic foot. Red and yellow dashed lines depict the marked mediolateral imbalance in foot/digit image on the left and the radiograph of the foot/digit on the right.

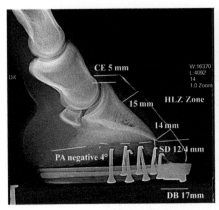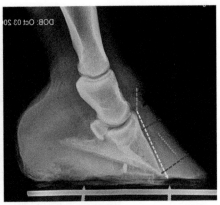

Fig. 11. There are several measured parameters that provide vital information and feedback to the farrier. When pathology and imbalance require specific mechanical realignment, it is vital that farriers know what they have to work with, specifically with the laminitic foot. The PA, sole depth, and digital breakover invariably are altered with every trim and shoe application. Green dotted line is the coronary extensor process distance; the red dotted lines represent the proximal and distal hoof-lamellar-zones; blue dotted line represents the normal angle of the hoof compared to the angle of rotation (yellow dotted line) of the third phalanx. Both images are of the 'Right foot'.

sink when the digit descends under load during ground contact in the stance phase. The ground-bearing support components consist of the digital cushion, ungual cartilage, frog, bars, sole, and ground-bearing surface wall. Understanding that a foot is balanced when the suspension and support components balanced and in equilibrium, equals a strategy for a therapeutic and maintenance plan for a healthy foot (**Fig. 12**).

Much of the biomechanics of the equine foot is subjective, debated, and unclear, despite the large quantity of new information relating to therapeutic shoeing techniques and distal limb biomechanics. Mechanics is the branch of science dealing with energy and forces and their effect on bodies and the functional parts involved in an activity; it requires measurable data that not always are available (**Fig. 13**).

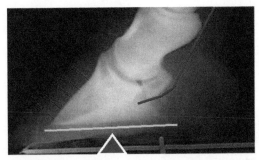

Fig. 12. A foot is balanced when the suspension and support components are in harmony and equilibrium and have total recall following deformation from load. Understanding the mechanics and forces at play greatly enhance the mechanical thought process as therapeutic or maintenance plans are strategized. Solid red line approximates the deep digital flexor tendon (DDFT), the thin red lines represent the hoof-lamellar zone distance, and the blue 'broken' line the position of the third phalanx when the foot is balanced. The red triangle represents the center of support for the foot.

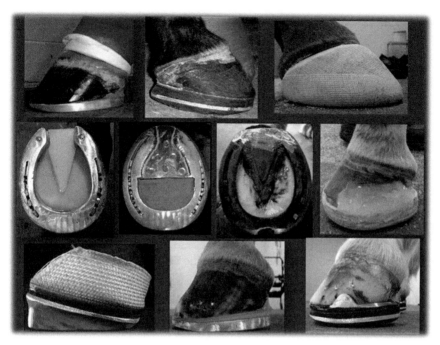

Fig. 13. Countless types of shoes and techniques have been developed and introduced for therapeutic or maintenance in an attempt to enhance functionality; the key is to become familiar with current understanding of how these applications work to biomechanical advantage.

Significance of the Influence of the Deep Digital Flexor Musculotendinous Unit

Proper tension in the DDFT is required for normal form and function of the equine digit whether at rest or motion. Given the hoof capsule is healthy and able to withstand the different forces placed on it, the DDFT improves and lessens capsular deformation and foot pathology. When 1 or more parts of the foot are exposed to poor genetics, repeated overload, injury, disease, environmental factors, or human intervention, however, an abnormal tension in the DDFT can worsen internal pathology and capsular distortion[23] (**Fig. 14**).

Perfusing the Foot Venograms

Radiographic contrast studies, referred to as *venograms*, can be helpful disclosing the relationship between load, laminae, sole corium, and vascular patency and may help to explain disparities in wall growth in the compromised digit[24] (**Fig. 15**). They clearly demonstrate the effect of the DDFT on the laminar attachment and thus on the hoof wall. If the limb is fully loaded during injection of the contrast agent, vessel filling of the laminar corium is constrained. Relieving tension in the DDFT by slight flexion of the carpus during the injection, however, permits normal filling of the laminar corium (**Fig. 16**). This finding implies that when the DDFT is under increased tension, so is the laminar attachment, in particular the dorsal hoof wall through the dermal-epidermal laminar connection to the horn of the wall. There is an interconnected network of structures involved: DDFT, P3, laminar attachment, solar corium, and

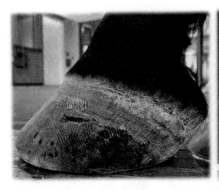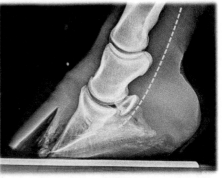

Fig. 14. When 1 or more components of the foot are subjected to ongoing, less-than-ideal parameters, the abnormal tension in the DDFT can cause or exacerbate internal pathology and capsular distortion. Dotted yellow line approximates the position of the deep digital flexor tendon (DDFT). Both images are of the 'Left foot'.

hoof capsule; therefore, when changing 1 part, the likely effects on the other structures should be considered.

Vessel Integrity

The venogram offers the first measurable evidence confirming laminitis, differentiating it from other diseases of the foot and before radiographs demonstrate clinical changes (**Fig. 17**). Previously, the only methods of diagnosing laminitis at the time of onset were history and clinical signs. These signs, however, are not pathognomonic for laminitis. Pain, once considered a good indicator to assess the rate severity of a laminitic event, also is an unreliable and repeatable indicator.

The venogram is a useful diagnostic tool that can demonstrate laminitic changes to vessels early in the disease. Venograms also can grade help the severity of the compromised blood flow and, therefore, provide a good diagnostic tool to identify acute cases of slight soreness (Obel grade 1 or less). Hooves that are nonreactive to pain after initial treatment do not equal hoof stability or resolution of the disease, and, if mistaken, can lead to poor mechanical support and treatment during the most important window of opportunity. Pain improvement does not equal resolution of the event because it does not

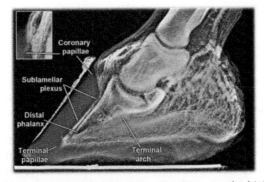

Fig. 15. Radiographic contrast studies, known as venograms, can be highly informative, to reveal the relationship between load, laminae, sole corium and vascular patency. (Image of a normal venogram courtesy Dr Amy Rucker.)

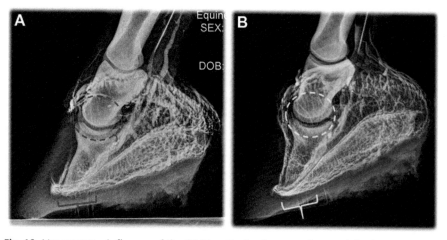

Fig. 16. Venograms—influence of the DDFT on the laminar attachment. (*A*) When the limb is fully loaded during injection of the contrast agent into the digital vein, vascular filling of the laminar corium is limited. (*B*) Relieving tension in the DDFT during dye injection allows normal filling of the laminar corium. Figure A, red circle, represents the 'stark loss of contrast of the coronary plexus extending to the dorsal aspect of the face of the coffin bone.' and the effect of contrast filling (red bracket) when the foot is loaded vs. figure B, yellow circle and bracket, when relieving tension on the deep digital flexor tendon (DDFT) and its effect on contrast filling in the venogram. Both radiographs are of the 'Left foot'.

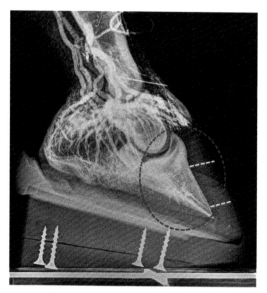

Fig. 17. The venogram provides the first detectable evidence that confirms laminitis, and reveals the damaging effects in the very early stages before radiographs present evidence of rotation and/or displacement of the coffin bone. Red circle is the area showing lack of filling of the vessels on the dorsal and ventral parts of the third phalanx when compared to a normal orientation of the hoof wall and third phalanx.

reflect the compromised state of reperfusion of the injured parts of the digit—key to defining an accurate prognosis. Subsequently, many horses progressively worsen during the first 6 weeks to 8 weeks after onset, simply because of a lack of recognition and the inability to minimize progressive injury and tissue degrading by not using proper mechanical reduction of DDFT tension, continuous monitoring of the state of vessel health, and continuing third phalanx displacement, until the disease is resolved. Comparative venograms are a more reliable means of assessing injury and prognosis if the blood supply fails to reestablish sufficient perfusion of the digit. Therefore, vessel reperfusion is a more meaningful representation of the term, *clinically stable*, than the overall pain response or radiographic findings.

Tenotomy Considerations

When a laminitic case remains clinically unresponsive to treatment, venograms can help in determining the need to perform a deep digital flexor (DDF) tenotomy to alleviate DDF forces contributing to lamellar and solar corium compression and compromised blood flow (**Fig. 18**). The importance of frequently monitoring a digit's blood supply, especially in the face of poor hoof/sole growth, is a good gauge of vascular health. In the acute, severe, nonresponsive cases, blood flow is compromised, and there is no noticeable improvement in horn/sole growth in the first 30 days to 45 days, even though employing DDF relief mechanical intervention. Waiting to triage the case, reliant on clinical progression before making decision for a DDF tenotomy, may result in irreversible damage, complications, and frequently humane euthanasia. The proactive approach often is lifesaving in high-risk cases involving laminitis.

Laminitis—Etiology

The etiology of laminitis is a secondary response to currently recognized primary triggers, such as endocrinopathic dysregulation, overloading–contralateral limb loading syndrome, and endotoxemia (please see Nora S. Grenager's article, "Endocrinopathic Laminitis," in this issue, Teresa A. Burns's article "'Feeding the

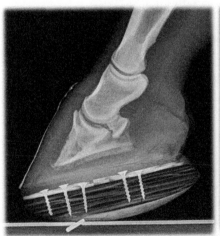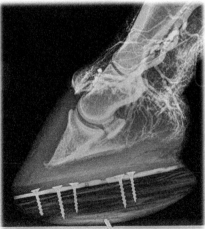

Fig. 18. Venograms can play a major assist to determine the need to perform DDF tenotomy because they can reveal clear evidence when the limits of the mechanical approach do not adequately relieve DDF forces at play that contribute to lamellar and solar coriuin compression with subsequent compromised blood flow. Both panels are of the 'Left foot'.

Foot': Nutritional Influences on Equine Hoof Health," in this issue, and Daniela Lue-thy's article, "Cryotherapy Techniques – Best Protocols to Support the Foot in Health and Disease," in this issue). Good progress continues to be made in better un-derstanding and treating this life-threatening disease of the horse.

Veterinarians and farriers often grapple with difficult treatment decisions, and the prognosis declines with increasing severity and repeated episodes of the disease. An initial poor prognosis, just by the diagnosis of laminitis, can improve by employing ur-gent emergency mechanical treatment (EMT). Laminitis can present with difficult and diverse clinical presentations as it develops through different stages and effects each horse differently because of dissimilar surviving mechanisms, including pain manifes-tation. Basing laminitis status solely on pain presentation may perpetuate a flawed conclusion that a horse is stable, that is, that acute pain cycle has subsided, with coffin bone displacement and distal descent and/or rotation, because of the laminitic event, with next steps centered on recovery support. Unfortunately, as discussed before, pain is not a predictable indicator of pathologic severity or recovery prognosis. In actuality, the main window of opportunity to relieve injury has closed considerably by the time displacement or distal descent is detected. Additionally, continued incremental injury follows if the series of events that perpetuated the lamellar insult remain undefined.

The EMT protocol is 2-fold; it requires (1) timely, purpose-driven accurate injury evaluation of the internal foot structures and (2) the viability of blood flow within the digit. This information is vital to completely comprehend the severity of the suspensory mechanism and the exact location(s) of blood vessel compromise in the foot. With an understanding of these important parameters, the clinician and farrier can optimize a plan for mechanical support for each digit. Simultaneously, the root cause of laminitis needs to be identified and solved, typically through medical, surgical, environmental, and nutritional intervention.

Several phases of laminitis have been categorized and recognized by the profes-sional community to describe the event.

The developmental phase occurs before clinical signs. It is the least understood and unnoticed, initiating a cascade of tissue injury. Although this phase is unobserved, lamellar injury is occurring and sets the stage for the acute phase.

The acute phase is indicated with the onset of clinical signs lasting 72 hours in duration and before third phalanx displacement occurs. The acute phase resolution varies relative to the effectiveness of mechanical and medical treatment. Starting preventive application of high-level hoof mechanics on day 1 of the acute phase can arrest or amazingly reduce the potential for displacement. Continued application of these mechanical aids, com-bined with medical treatment and continued monitoring over multiple cycles, is essential to prevent relapsing, until hoof stability is regained. Although horses respond positively to anti-inflammatory drugs and mechanical relief with improved signs of comfort, reduction in pain during the first few days to weeks does not indicate laminitic resolution, so strict confinement is required because unnecessary movement increases the forces working on the weakened parts and further destabilizes the hoof capsule. Besides restriction of movement, in a confined area or stall with deep bedding, it is important to control forces on the digit. During this time, laminitic horses may experience acute spontaneous lame-ness due to sequestra of necrotic corium and/or bone necrosis that manifests as an ab-scess. Dependent on severity of instability, these changes may continue for 6 weeks to 8 weeks as the digit moves toward the chronic phase (**Fig. 19**).

The chronic phase has been described as the later phase of a laminitic episode once displacement has occurred with hoof wall deformity. At this point in time, the digit needs 8 months to 10 months to regrow a new hoof capsule from coronet to weight-bearing surface, with improved stability. When proactive measures are implemented, there may be little detectable displacement, the end point being a well-managed chronic compensated case (**Fig. 20**).

The chronic uncompensated case is more guarded in the prognosis due to considerable irreversible, soft tissue and bone injury that is clinically evident with hoof distortions and avulsions. Many of these cases suffer from recurrent abscesses, necrotic bone degeneration and resorption, necrotic hoof wall avulsion, and severe contraction of the deep and superficial flexor tendons (**Fig. 21**).

Vascular Compromise

The severity of the initial laminitic episode and subsequent compromised vascular perfusion determine the level of cellular destruction to the lamellar interface and the intricate support that fixes the coffin bone to hoof wall. With the bone/hoof bond interface compromised, flexor forces acting on the laminae and bone increase the likelihood of displacement or sinking/dropping of the coffin bone. Therefore, it is vital to facilitate reperfusion before the domino effect of vascular deficiency injures important components of the suspensory apparatus and horn growth centers. Efficient EMT used as a standard preventive mediation can help avoid or minimize lamellar loss by decreasing vascular compression and compensation (**Fig. 22**). The DDF unit plays an important role in disrupting the coffin bone alignment once the dorsal lamellar interface is weakened from the inflammation of laminitis. The lamellar interface no longer is resilient enough to maintain suspension and normal positioning of the coffin bone. Without neutralizing actions to compensate for the impaired lamellar tissue, the DDFT, because of its P3 insertion and unopposed flexor moments, may rotate the coffin bone, causing compression of the sensitive solar corium and circumflex artery. The compromised blood flow affects foot growth and healing. A lamellar wedge creates mechanical forces that precludes better lamellar/horn connections derived from the coronet wall growth center. Therefore, reperfusion of essential tissues takes precedence.

The intensity and period of vascular compromise to the solar rim affect the outcome of most cases. When the circumflex vessels are prolapsed, stripping the apex of P3 of its blood supply, bone resorbs, causing a distinctive edge that can be seen on the lateral radiograph. Thus, adequate perfusion to the bone margins is needed to preserve bone integrity and prevent osteolysis (**Fig. 23**).

Therapeutic Approaches Using Mechanical Principles

The main goal, in using mechanical principals to treat laminitis, is to neutralize the mechanical forces that that compromise lamellae and corium vessels as soon as

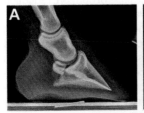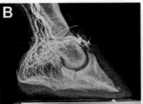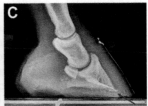

Fig. 19. (A) The acute phase has been suggested to be the onset of clinical signs lasting 72 hours in duration and or before displacement occurs. (B) Depending on severity of instability, this morphing may continue up to 6 weeks to 8 weeks as the digit moves toward the chronic phase. (C) Horses may experience acute spontaneous lameness due to sequestrae of necrotic corium and/or bone necrosis that manifest as abscesses (red arrow).

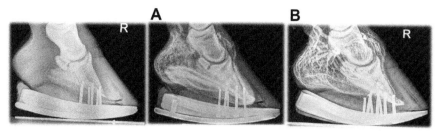

Fig. 20. Comparative venograms are a more reliable means of assessing the extent of the damage and potential prognosis. (*A*) Vascular patency is a more meaningful representation of the severity of the condition, (*B*) restoring perfusion in the digit over time with adequate mechanical aid. 'Left panel is lateral-medial view of right foot before venogram study in A and B.

possible. Applying the Modified Ultimate (NANRIC, Lawrenceburg, KY) or a similar support that approaches a 20° ground PA with improved breakover is the first step in the emergency mechanical treatment (EMT) protocol (**Fig. 24**). An elevation between 15° and 20° PA is necessary to sufficiently diminish the pulling forces of the DDFT/muscle unit working on the unstable dorsal laminae/coffin bone interface. Research and practical experience show that an elevation of approximately 20° PA and ideal toe breakover greatly reduce rotational forces on bone and downward tension on the coffin bone tip. Heel elevation lessens bone compression of the corium and dislocation of the circumflex artery, minimizing vascular loss and its associate pain. With proper DDFT counteraction at disease onset, rotation seldom occurs. In cases of DDFT contraction persisting and vascular compromise continuing, despite using the EMT protocol, DDF tenotomy may be needed (**Fig. 25**).

Deep Digital Flexor Tenotomy

Pre-tenotomy and Post-tenotomy hoof preparation is important for successful results. Before the tenotomy, a derotation trim (ground parallel PA) is performed followed by a mechanical 15° to 20° elevation of PA, to create tendon laxity to enable the surgical procedure (**Fig. 26**). Transecting the tendon relieves tension on weakened dorsal

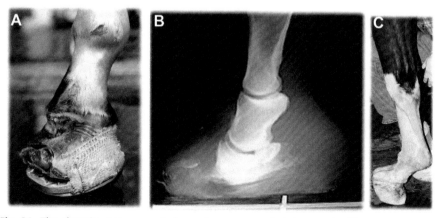

Fig. 21. The chronic uncompensated case is more guarded due to significant irreversible, soft tissue and bone damage. Many of these cases suffer from (*A*) recurrent abscesses, (*B*) necrotic bone degeneration and resorption, (*C*) and severe contraction of the deep and superficial flexor tendons.

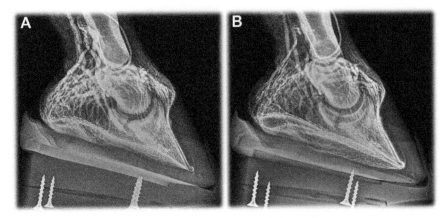

Fig. 22. Efficient EMT applied as a standard preventive intervention can help avoid or minimize lamellar damage by minimizing vascular compression and compensation. Use of a reliable, repeatable damage assessment protocol is paramount to effectively treat and monitor the vascular and tissue response. (*A*) First day of mechanical aid application; (*B*) 3 days post-reperfusion to vital tissues is priority.

laminae, increasing blood flow to the secondary laminae and decompressing sensitive solar fimbria, promoting increased sole growth (**Fig. 27**). This desired growth pattern offers a better long-term prognosis. Post-tenotomy, the heel elevation/PA is meticulously lowered by removing the wedges and creating a separation between the incised tendon ends, providing the needed time for realignment of the phalanges and reestablishment of vessel health before the tendon heals. Trimming post-tenotomy is to maintain the alignment of P3 and hoof wall (**Fig. 28**).

The low-profile foot often develops more toe than heel growth and has a persistent negative PA that requires radiographs to assist in corrective trimming and/or shoeing (**Fig. 29**). The upright foot profile foot invariably is more challenging and has a stronger predisposition for contracture, bone necrosis, and large bone resorption (**Fig. 30**).

Scar tissue contracture after a DDF tenotomy is a potential sequala. Widespread bone resorption and remodeling of hard and soft tissues can trigger secondary mechanoreceptors that stimulate the contracture reflex (pain contracture) despite an initial

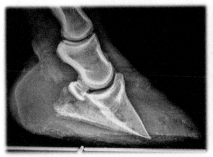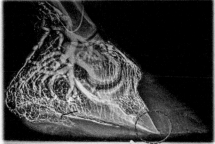

Fig. 23. The degree and duration period of vascular compromise to the solar rim influences the outcome of most cases. It is imperative that adequate perfusion be reestablished to the bone to preserve bone integrity and mitigate bone lysis. Red dotted circle represents the area devoid of contrast material on venogram. Both panels are of the 'Right foot'.

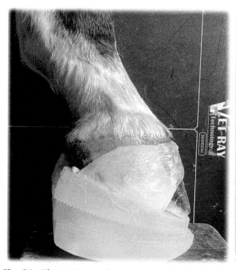
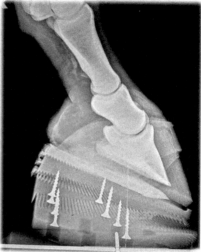

Fig. 24. The main goal in using mechanical principals for treating the ill effects of laminitis is to reverse the mechanical component that is diminishing patency of the lamellae and corium vessels as soon as possible. Applying the Modified Ultimate or a similar aid that offers a 20° ground PA with enhanced breakover is the first step of the emergency protocol. Both panels are of the 'Right foot'. end (NANRIC, Lawrenceburg, KY).

favorable response. Performing the tenotomy when bone disease is radiographically evident can produce favorable results; however, many relapse and contract, increasing the PA and overloading the solar corium. The cycle of pain contracture is enhanced when imprudent efforts are made to control the PA by lowering the heels too soon, causing premature increased DDFT engagement (**Fig. 31**).

There are several questions to consider when making the decision to perform a DDF tenotomy: degree/severity of injury, short-term and long-term goals of the owner,

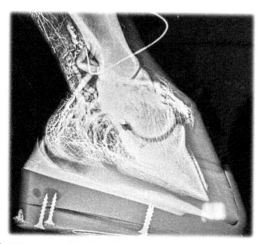

Fig. 25. In cases of DDFT contraction that is unresponsive and vascular compromise is non-resolved using conventional mechanical treatment, DDF tenotomy may prove beneficial.

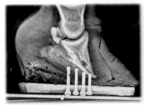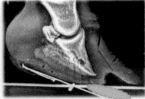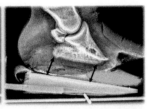

Fig. 26. Transection of the DDFT allow immediate realignment of the coffin bone relative to the ground surface. Prior to the tenotomy, a derotation trim (ground parallel PA) is performed. Red dashed lines represent the trim line parallel to the PA of the coffin bone. Yellow lines represent the shoe placement parallel to the PA of the coffin bone. Green circle represent the impression material derotating the hoof capsule allowing the shoe and coffin bone angle to have a 0 degree Capsule PA. The blue lines depicts the same distance of and ideal 20 mm sole depth between the wings and tip of the coffin bone achievng a derotated coffin paralel to the shoe.

aftercare experience of responsible personnel, mechanical understanding and skill level of the farrier and veterinarian, and financial considerations. Young horses do well post-tenotomy, often returning to normal function, whereas older horses are less likely to return to normal function. A well-planned strategy plan improves the outcome and success of tenotomy cases (**Fig. 32**).

Concluding Remarks

Laminitis remains an insidious high-risk health and welfare problem of the horse. Although important advances in understanding the mechanisms of this disease have been made, it is not possible to effectively prevent the disease and repair injured lamellar tissue. There are many ways to treat laminitis; however, the best window of

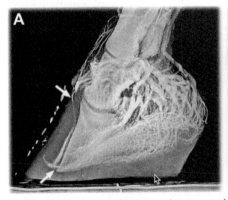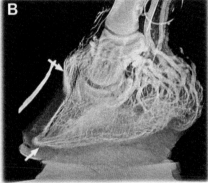

Fig. 27. DDF tentomy releases tension on weak dorsal laminae increasing blood flow to secondary laminae and decompressing sensitive solar terminal papillae to promote vascular reperfiision and increased sole growth. (*A*) Pre-DDF tenotomy. (*Arrows*) Compromised vascular supply of the coronary plexus and dorsal displacement of the circumflex vessel occluding the solar plexus. (*B*) Post-DDF tenotomy. Evidence of vascular reperfusion of the previous compromised areas. (Images courtesy of Dr Amy Rucker.). Figure A is a venogram pre-DDFT tenotomy with arrows showing lack of vessel filling on venogram, and figure B is the comparison post DDFT tenotomy.

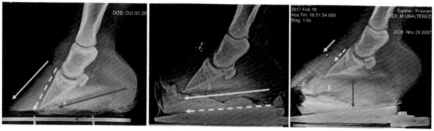

Fig. 28. Subsequent trims post-tenotomy maintain the alignment and post-farriery attention to detail often dictate the successful outcome of the procedure. (Courtesy of Dr. Ric Redden).

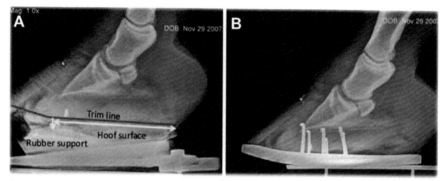

Fig. 29. The low-profile foot often develops more toe growth than heel and has a persistent negative PA that requires radiographic-assisted collective trim and/or shoeing. (*A*) Preshoeing strategic plan with accomplished goals confirmed (*B*) postshoeing. (Courtesy of Dr. Ric Redden).

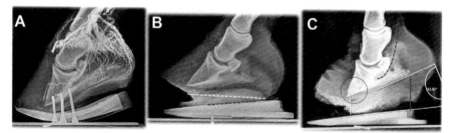

Fig. 30. The steeper profile foot invariably is more problematic and as a rule has a much stronger tendency to redevelop a contracture with accumulative bone necrosis and extensive resorption. (*A*) Venogram with evidence of severe vascular deficits despite the attempts of different mechanical aids. (*B*) Derotation shoe post-DDF tenotomy achieving a parallel alignment with the shoe (Red dotted line represents the alignment of the third phalanx and shoe after DDFT tenotomy and the yellow line the position of the third phalanx relative to the ground surface). (*C*) Scar tissue constrictive have tendency of increasing the PA and once again loading the solar corium with accumulative bone necrosis and extensive resorption. The yellow dashed line outlines the most distal aspect of the hoof capsule / sole. Everything distal is the impression material maintaing hoof capsule postion aligning the derotated coffin bone paralel to the shoe (red dashed lines).

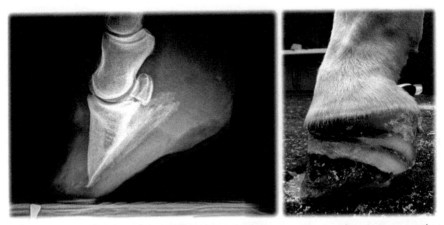

Fig. 31. Bone resorption and remodeling can trigger secondary mechano-receptors that stimulate the contracture reflex (pain contracture). This cycle of pain contracture is accelerated when misguided efforts are made to control the PA by lowering the heels too soon causing premature increased DDFT engagement. Both panels are of the 'Left foot'.

opportunity is at the beginning. Once rotation and infection occur, the prognosis for full recovery is guarded. Although there is a direct relationship between the severity of disease and it is accompanying pathology, there is a small window of opportunity to alleviate some of the destructive effects, and thus proactive measures is the best medicine.

Sheared heels

Heel problems tend to be reoccurring because the primary problem never was corrected. Knowing the etiology of a foot problem helps formulate a successful treatment plan for healing, preventing reoccurrence and improving the welfare and well-being of the horse. A common problem is the reoccurring quarter crack, which rarely occurs without being preceded by hoof capsule distortion, referred to as *shunted heel*, *sheared heel*, or *displaced heel* (**Fig. 33**).

Shunted heels occur because 1 heel is overloaded more than the other, causing it to displace in an upward direction. As the heel bulb and heel hoof wall and quarter regions are displaced proximally, the wall reaches a tipping point in its elasticity, causing the heel to crack at the hairline, and a bleeding, painful quarter crack. If the heel remains in the shunted position, the foot is at increased risk of cracking again. Sheared heels are thought to be the result of a conformational defect causing overloading of 1 part of the foot, for example, the medial (inside) heel of a front foot and, in the pelvic limbs, and laterally also. The predisposing conformation recognized as a risk factor for shunted medial heels is outward rotation of the thoracic limbs (**Fig. 34**).

Most horses with outward rotation move poorly with a winging in gait. This causes limb interference and therefore rarely are elite athletes. Between the years 2010 and 2014, 72 sheared heels in Thoroughbreds were clinically evaluated and photographed for conformation. Radiographs of the feet were taken from the front and side to assess foot balance. Of the 72 sheared heels on front feet, 70 sheared heels were medial and 2 were lateral. Both cases of lateral sheared heels had a fetlock varus conformation. Of the 70 medial sheared heels, 60 had a combination of carpal valgus and inward

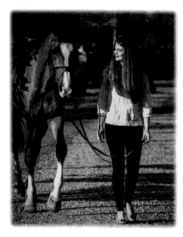
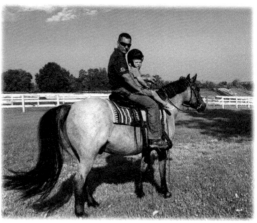

Fig. 32. A well-made strategic plan will improve the outcome and success of many of these tenotomy cases. Both panels are equine patients after recovery from 'Deep digital flexor tenotomy for treatment of chronic laminitis'.

rotation of the distal limb conformation, 8 had the classic outward rotation of the limb, 1 had fetlock valgus, and 1 had normal conformation (no major conformation fault).

Using radiographs, the relationship of medial to lateral imbalance and sheared heels was investigated. Vertical distance from the medial and lateral wings of the pedal bone to the ground surface was measured on standard horizontal front views of front feet, and

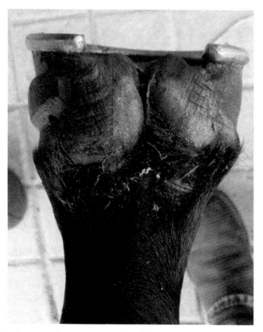

Fig. 33. Shunted heels occur because 1 side of the heel is loaded more than the other, causing it to displace upward. Red dotted line represents the difference in heels with overloading of one heel more than another.

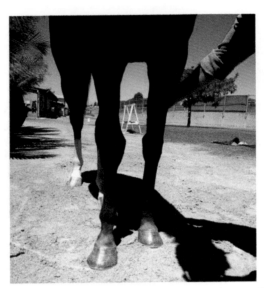

Fig. 34. The conformation that has historically been recognized to predispose the shunted medial heels is outward rotation of the front limbs.

significant difference between the normal and sheared heel cases was able to be detected. The sheared heel feet were out of balance medial to lateral, with the medial heel being lower (**Figs. 35–37**) (Morrison, Beasley, and Morell, unpublished data, 2015).

The most common conformation that predisposes to a sheared heel is carpal valgus and inward rotation of the digit. The rotation usually occurs because of a spiral deformity of the metacarpus (cannon) or pastern bone. As the digit rotates inward, it places the medial heel bulb directly below the boney column or vertical line of force (**Fig. 38**). The medial heel bulb, therefore, bears a greater loading force, causing it to collapse inward and shunted upward.

Because the medial wall is overloaded, the vessels are compressed, affecting normal hoof wall and sole growth on the medial side of the foot. As medial hoof growth slows, other regions of the foot maintain normal growth, resulting in a hoof imbalance with a lower medial hoof wall and further inward rotation of the digit. Previous studies report that as the medial hoof is lowered or the lateral part of the hoof raised, the digit rotates inward causing a cycle of overload imbalance and additional overload.[13]

Management of the shunted heel

There are several effective foot strategies to treat this problem; the first is the trim. The hoof needs to be trimmed for balance, symmetric DIP joint space, and uniform sole depth supporting the pedal bone. As discussed previously, the shunted heel usually is lower on the shunted heel side, and, therefore, the feet need to be lowered on the side opposite the shunted heel (**Figs. 39 and 40**). The goal is to trim the foot so that the solar surface is perpendicular to the long axis of the pastern; a "T" square can be used to establish the proper trim when radiographs are not available.

The second component of effective treatment is support, provided in several ways. A frog support bar, pad, or stabilizer plate is an effective way to give frog support and to redistribute weight away from the hoof capsule in the heel region (**Fig. 41**). These clinical cases get some immediate benefit from floating or unweighting the affected heel by creating a space between the ground surface of the hoof and the shoe (a

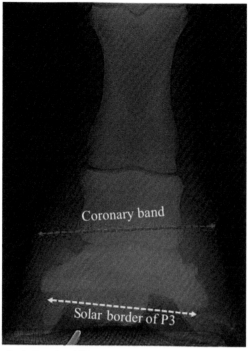

Fig. 35. Radiograph depicting the difference in lateral to medial angles with overloading of one heel more than another.

non–weight-bearing region below the displaced coronary band and heel bulb), allowing the shunted heel to settle or drop.

Shunted heel cases should be trimmed and reshod every 3 weeks to 4 weeks. Because the hoof grows unevenly, the imbalance is greatest toward the end of each shoeing cycle and at increased risk of injury; most quarter cracks occur toward the end of the shoeing cycle. With careful management and special attention to the precipitating factors for sheared heels, many quarter cracks and sheared heels can be

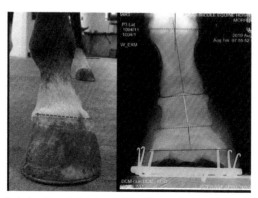

Fig. 36. Left panel (left foot) and right panel (radiograph of left foot) depicting the asymmetry in lateral to medial balance with overloading of one heel more than another. Both panels are of the 'Left front foot'.

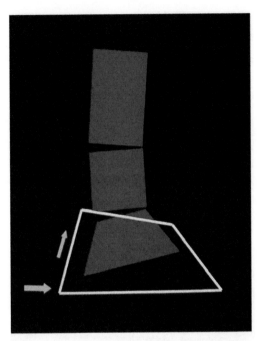

Fig. 37. Representative model of lateral to medial imbalance in foot/digit and goal in trimming to compensate for the marked imbalance (green arrows and white outline of hoof).

prevented (**Fig. 42**). The aforementioned case was also treated with sub coronary band grooving. A procedure in which a horizontal groove is made below the coronary band. This technique is thought to make the hoof wall more pliable, allowing the displaced coronary band ti settle or drop down.

PROPHYLACTIC SHOEING TECHNIQUES—MINIMIZING STRESS IN THE UPPER-LEVEL PERFORMANCE HORSE

The importance of foot shape and balance is vital in maintaining soundness and performance in the upper-level equine athlete. Functionally adapted for speed and efficient use of energy, the foot is quite light weight compared with the large mass it supports and a common source of lameness in equine athlete. Estimates are that the heel region of the foot accounts for greater than one-third of chronic lameness in the horse and the only part of the horse's body in continuous contact with the ground, equaling more trauma and injury. Studies report a healthy foot can dampen the ground vibrations on impact by as much as 80% to 90%.[25]

A well-developed hoof capsule, with appropriate mass, shape, and moisture content, is the foundation for a normal functioning foot. Several mechanisms are in place to help shock absorption: (1) hoof wall; (2) lamellar interface; (3) soft tissue (joint, joint capsule, sole corium, digital cushion, tendon/ligament, and bone); and (4) movement of blood into and out of the foot.

When the foot is loaded, the elastic hoof capsule deforms, soft tissues are compressed and stretched, and the elastic/malleable lamellar interface allows the boney column to displace slightly within the hoof capsule.

As the foot is loaded, the compression and tension within the foot squeeze the blood out of the foot and help drive the blood up the limb via low-resistance vascular pathways

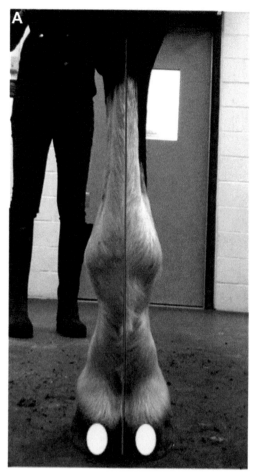 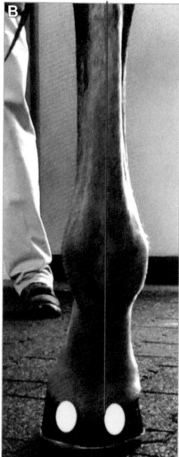

Fig. 38. (A) Normal conformation; (B) inward rotation of the distal limb. Both panels are of the 'Right thoracic limb'.

in the collateral cartilages. The anatomic parts responsible for translating external shock into movement of blood are the bars, digital cushion, and collateral cartilages. It has been theorized that as the heels impact the ground, the bars receive vibrations and forces, which then convey the vibrations and forces to the collateral cartilages, which lie deep to the bars.[26] The collateral cartilages are rich in blood vessels, containing a pool of blood, converting the vibrations into the movement of fluid/blood up the limb. Basically, the collateral cartilage and its blood vessels provide a low-resistance pathway for the rapid movement of blood from the foot during ground impact and act as a hydraulic shock absorber. Feet that are effective at shock absorption have thick, healthy collateral cartilages (with abundant blood supply), well-developed digital cushion, and strong established bars[27] (**Fig. 43**).

Feet need proper form to function properly, which simply means that the anatomic structures are of proper mass and spatial arrangement to execute the sequence of events needed to accommodate the dispersal of vibrations generated during ground impact and simultaneously supporting the weight of the horse. There are several goals to promote a healthy and well-functioning hoof. (1) The center of rotation (**Fig. 44** red

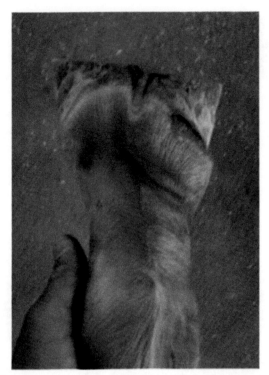

Fig. 39. View of foot/digit unweighted showing marked lateral to medial imbalance of heels.

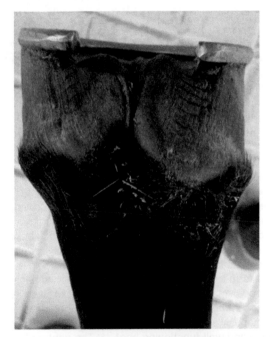

Fig. 40. Unweighted view of foot/digit of a less severe lateral to medial imbalance before trimming and reshoeing.

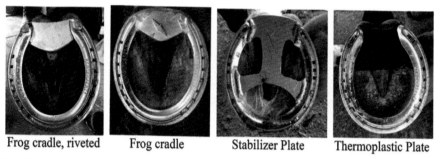

Frog cradle, riveted   Frog cradle   Stabilizer Plate   Thermoplastic Plate

Fig. 41. A frog support bar, pad, or stabilizer plate is an effective way to give frog support and to redistribute weight away from the hoof capsule in the heel region.

dot) lines up with the center of the weight-bearing surface of the foot. The center of rotation is easily identified, because it usually corresponds to the widest part of the sole. (2) A positive PA (blue line), between 2° and 5°, should be established. (3) A sole depth equaling the thickness of the horn lamellar zone (HLZ), (fig.44 yellow lines). The HLZ is the distance from the parietal surface of the pedal bone to the external surface of the hoof wall. (4) The heel position should be at the widest part of the frog **(Fig. 44)**.

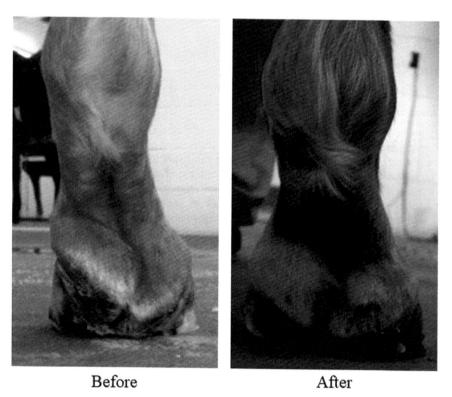

Before   After

Fig. 42. Before and after photos depicts a sheared heel on a barrel horse before and after treatment with proper trimming and frog support. This case also received subcoronary band grooving. Both panels are of the 'Right front foot'. Both panels are of the 'Right front foot'.

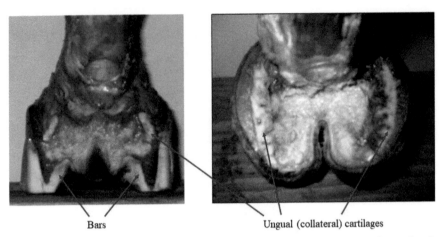

Bars   Ungual (collateral) cartilages

Fig. 43. Collateral cartilage and its blood vessels provide a low-resistance pathway for the rapid movement of blood from the foot during ground impact and act as a hydraulic shock absorber.

An under-run heel, where the heels are shifted forward, creates a situation where the bars and collateral cartilages are not aligned and cannot absorb shock as well as a foot with well-positioned heels and lines up with the collateral cartilages (**Fig. 45**). Part A of **Fig. 45** is an example of a well-balanced foot with ideal heel position and normal proportions to the weight-bearing structures of the foot. Parts C and D of **Fig. 45** are feet with under-run heels. The weight-bearing portion of the heel is tubules drift forward and no longer lines up with the shock absorbing mechanisms of the foot.

Causes of Under-run Heels

Arches and straight lines are strong architectural shapes, and strong feet have a sole arch and straight walls. Viewing the foot from the coronary band, the wall should be straight without flares or dishes. When feet are overloaded and distorted, the sole arch typically flattens and the wall bends or flares, creating a distortion. Distortions are a result of either overloading a healthy structure, causing it to collapse or bend, or it can be the result of underloading a structure, for example, a contracted heel on a clubfoot. In these cases, the heel is underloaded and the toe is overloaded, causing the heel to contract and the toe to bend or dish. Most upper-level athletes stress the heel region of the foot, which lowers the heel over time.[28] As the angle PA decreases, more force is placed on the heel, creating a vicious cycle that is difficult to correct. The heel region of the hoof is softer and more pliable than the toe because it is designed to dispel shock. The heel encloses the collateral cartilages, digital cushion, and an abundant vascular system, all designed to absorb shock. The toe is more rigid and designed to pierce the ground for traction. Because the heel is more malleable and hits the ground first, hoof distortions typically present here first.

A common hoof capsule distortion is the under-run heel believed to be caused by the process of shoeing and where normal hoof wear is prevented. The hoof wall grows in length during the normal shoeing cycle, with increasing toe length and decreasing hoof wall angle over time. As the toe grows, it shifts the heels forward and, with repeated trimming and rebalancing over multiple cycles, the horn tubules drift forward. Another shoeing consideration is the change in the foot's loading pattern; in the un-shod foot, the load is distributed to the sole, bars, frog, and hoof wall, whereas in

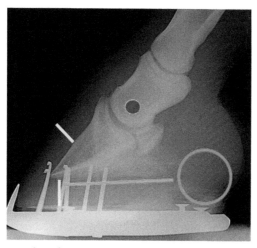

Fig. 44. There are several goals to promote a healthy and well-functioning hoof. (1) The center of rotation (*red dot*) lines up with the center of the weight-bearing surface of the foot. The center of rotation easily is identified, because usually it corresponds to the widest part of the sole. (2) Establishing a positive PA (*blue line*), between 2° and 5°. (3) A sole depth equaling the thickness of the HLZ thickness (*yellow lines*). (4) The heel position (green circle) should be at the widest part of the frog. HLZ, hoof lamellar zone.

the shod foot, the load is focused primarily on the hoof wall. The shod foot in soft footing, however, incorporates the sole, bars, and frog into weight bearing.

Important factors in preventing a compromised heel from occurring are maintaining ideal weight-bearing proportions to the weight-bearing surface of the foot and recognizing a vulnerable heel and treating it before a lameness occurs. An early morphologic sign of an overloaded heel is a frog that begins to prolapse or break the plane of the solar surface of the hoof wall (**Fig. 46**). The wall in the heel region begins to collapse or recede as it is overloaded, and the frog plane becomes lower than the hoof wall. Another sign of excessive heel concussion are hairs that begin to rise, and there is a dermatitis of the heel bulbs (**Fig. 47**).

The most effective way to repair a weakened or compromised heel is to go barefoot for a period. The frog plane improves, and the under-run heel position corrects rapidly when the horse is left barefoot. Frequently, this treatment option is not possible requiring shoes to maintain soundness for training and competition. In these cases,

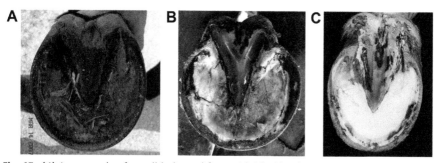

Fig. 45. (*A*) An example of a well-balanced foot with ideal heel position and normal proportions to the weight-bearing structures of the foot. (*B, C*) Feet with under-run heels.

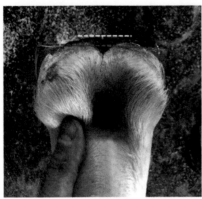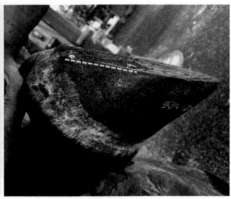

Fig. 46. Morphologic signs of an overloaded heel is a frog that begins to prolapse or break the plane of the solar surface of the hoof wall. The wall in the heel region begins to collapse or recede as it is overloaded, and the frog plane becomes lower than the hoof wall. Left panel (palmar/plantar view) - yellow dotted line represents the position of the frog in relation to the hoof wall (red dotted line). Right panel- relationship of the frog (red dotted line) in relation to hoof wall (yellow dotted line) on lateral view of the foot.

shoeing methods, simulating the barefoot condition, are required to rehabilitate the heel. **Fig. 48** is a race filly's foot before and after being barefoot for 3 months. The most effective way to repair a weakened or compromised heel is to go barefoot for a period. Several features of the barefoot condition, which can be replicated with shoeing to create a similar effect include frog support, rolled heel, rolled toe, and broad toe shape.

When evaluating a healthy barefoot, it should be noticed that the foot is not completely flat—the heels and the toe are rolled slightly. The rolled heel decreases excessive concussion generated during heel first landing. The rolled toe decreases resistance to breakover and allows the foot to rollover in any direction that is less stressful for that limb's conformation. The rolled heels give the ability to improve the heel position, by trimming the heels to the widest part of the frog without penetrating the sole underneath the wing of the third phalanx (**Fig. 49**). Horses need as much protection under the wing of the third phalanx, a common point of tenderness in athletes. If the entire foot is trimmed level, and the heels trimmed to the widest part of the frog, it means too much sole depth under the third phalanx is removed. Another part of rehabilitating the heel is frog support best done using a heart bar, frog cradle, stabilizer plate, frog support pad, or a temporary orthotic/sole support.

The Clubfoot

The clubfoot has strong heel structures and plenty of heel mass and can be a source of chronic heel pain. The clubfoot overloads the toe and the boney column, causing the common pathologies of arthritis, sidebones, pedal osteitis of the apex of the P3, navicular bone sclerosis, osteoarthritis, and contracted heels. The compressive forces on the navicular bone are increased as the DDFT is pulled tighter along the flexor surface of the navicular bone. It has been demonstrated that upright or clubfeet have a thinner fibrocartilage layer compared with normal feet and likely a result of the increased compressive forces of the DDFT against the flexor surface of the navicular bone. Clubfeet often have increased wall growth in the heels and slower wall growth at the toe, as the foot attempts to raise the heels and unload or accommodate the contracted DDFT,

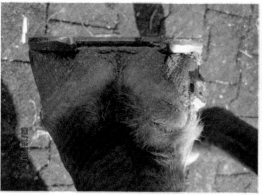
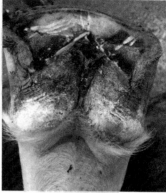

Fig. 47. Other signs of excessive heel concussion are hairs that begin to rise and dermatitis of the heel bulbs.

and the foot remodels to accommodate all phases of the stride. Because the DDFT is under the most tension just before heel lift off (break over), it is this phase of the stride that must be addressed when rebalancing the clubfoot. Substantially enhancing/easing break over and trimming the heels to a more normal height allow these feet to return to normal. **Fig. 50** depicts the same clubfoot after several shoeing cycles to accommodate the contracted DDFT.

Most clubfeet can achieve equal toe/heel growth and resolve the anterior dish with these simple mechanics. It is important to understand that the contracture is not being fixed or resolved but merely accommodated with simple shoeing mechanics, allowing the foot to return to a normal shape, with even wall growth, no dish, good anterior sole

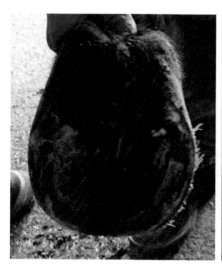
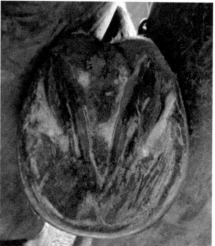

Before   After

Fig. 48. illustrates a race filly's foot before and after being barefoot for 3 months. Notice the improved heel position, weight-bearing proportions, and overall shape of the foot.

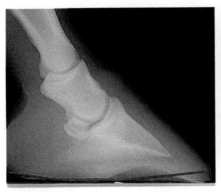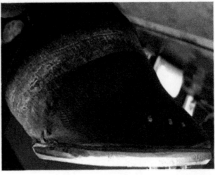

Fig. 49. The rolled heels give the ability to improve the heel position, by trimming the heels to the widest part of the frog without penetrating the sole underneath the wing of the third phalanx. Both panels are of the 'Right front foot'.

depth, therefore, a stronger, healthier foot. High-speed video and gait analysis studies are needed to better understand how the clubfoot responds to the shoeing. It is posited that clubfoot horses do not have to take a short step to accommodate the tendon in the caudal phase of the stride because, when the break over is reduced, they lengthen the caudal phase and consequently take a longer stride. The other possibility is that they are more comfortable in this type of shoe and change their gait accordingly. When evaluating and treating a lower limb lameness, which may be secondary to the tendon contracture, the first step should be to address hoof distortion or to rebalance the clubfoot by trimming the heels and moving the breakover beneath the anterior coronary band. This alleviates the tendon contracture to some degree and allows the foot to function more normally foot and, frequently, the secondary lameness resolves or greatly improves. As the affected foot loads the heels, heel contracture tends to improve with time and use. In cases of frog atrophy, loading the frog, sulci, and bars with an elastic impression material stimulates and loads these structures. These feet often benefit from having the foot's shock absorbing structures engaged or stimulated with a soft and elastic sole support material.

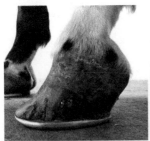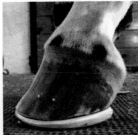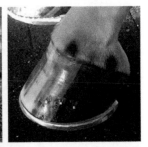

Fig. 50. Substantially enhancing/easing break over and trimming the heels to a more normal height allows these feet to return to normal. This figure depicts the same clubfoot after several shoeing cycles to accommodate the contracted DDFT. Left figure is a club foot before 1st trimming; middle figure is after several trimmings; and right panel is the final appearance of the foot.

CLINICS CARE POINTS

- Parameters measured on radiographs include sole depth, phalangeal alignment, palmer/plantar angle, HLZ/dorsal hoof wall thickness, bone angle, CED, angle of flexor surface of navicular bone, center of rotation, center of articulation, joint spacing, dorsal hoof wall hoof angle, and heel angle.

- The DDFT plays a major role in forces on the digit via its musculotendon unit. The DDFT forces on the coffin bone are neutralized by opposing forces of healthy laminae/bone/horn and, to a lesser extent, by the forces of the extensor tendon.

- The venogram is a useful diagnostic tool demonstrating laminitic vessel changes early in the disease and help grade the severity of the compromised blood flow. The venogram is a good diagnostic tool in identifying acute cases of slight soreness (Obel grade 1 or less).

- The DDF unit plays an important role in disrupting the coffin bone alignment once the dorsal lamellar interface is weakened from laminitis. With proper DDFT neutralization at disease onset, rotation seldom occurs; however, if DDFT contraction persists and vascular compromise continues, despite using the EMT protocol, DDF tenotomy likely is needed.

- Heel problems reoccur if the primary problem is not corrected. Understanding the cause of the foot problem aides in formulating a successful treatment plan for healing, prevention, and improving the soundness and well-being of the horse.

REFERENCES

1. Balch O, White K and Butler D. How lameness is associated with selected aspects of hoof imbalance. Proc 39 Annual convention American association of equine practitioners 1993.
2. Anderson TM, McIlwraith CW, Douay P. The role of conformation in musculoskeletal problems in the racing thoroughbred. Equine Vet J 2004;36:571–5.
3. Eliashar E, McGuigan M, Wilson A. Relationship of foot conformation and force applied to the navicular bone of sound horses at the trot. Equine Vet J 2004; 36:431–5.
4. Kane A, Stover S, Gardner I, et al. Hoof size, shape, and balance as possible risk factors for catastrophic musculoskeletal injury of thoroughbred racehorses. Am J Vet Res 1998;59(12):1545–52.
5. Viitanen MJ, Wilson AM, McGuigan HP, et al. Effect of hoof balance on the intra-articular pressure in the distal interpha- langeal joint in vitro. Equine Vet J 2003; 35:184–9.
6. Kate Holroyd a, Jonathon J, Dixon b, et al. Variation in foot conformation in lame horses with different foot lesions. Vet J 2013 Mar;195(3):361–5.
7. Value of quality foot radiographs and their impact on practical Farriery Randy B. Eggleston, AAEP Procedings 2012 Vol. 58
8. Frederik E. Pauwels, Chris W. Rogers, Heather Wharton, Radiographic measurements of hoof balance are significantly influenced by a horse's stance, Vet Radiol Ultrasound 2017;58(1). p. 10-17
9. Balch O, Butler D, Collie M. Balancing the normal foot: hoof preparation, shoe fit and shoe modification in the performance horse. Equine Uet Educ 1997;9(3): 143–54.
10. Wilson AM, McGuigan MP, Fouracre L, et al. The force and contact stress on the navicular bone during trot locomotion in sound horses and horses with Navicular disease. Equine Vet J 2001;33:159–65.
11. Clayton H. The effect of an acute hoof wall angulation on the stride kinematics of trotting horses. Equine Vet J Suppl 1990;9:86–90.

12. Oosterlinck M, Pille F, Huppes T, Gasthuyes F. Back W Comparison of pressure plate and force plate gait kinetics in sound Warmbloods at walk and trot. Vet J 2010 Dec;186(3):347–51.

13. Chateau H, Degueurce C Jerbik H, Crevier-denoix N, et al. Three-dimensional kinematics of the equine interphalangeal joints: articular impact of asymmetric bearing. Vet Res 2002;33:371–82.

14. Tekscan, Inc. 307 West First Street South Boston,MA 02127 info@tekscan.com

15. Werkman Black, Helper Molenstraat 43, 9721 BT Groningen The Netherlands, black@werkmanhoofcare.com

16. Meriam JG. The role and importance of farriery in equine veterinary practice. Vet Clin North Am 2003;19:273–83.

17. Pauwels F, Rogers C, Wharton H, et al. Radiographic measurements of hoof balance are significantly influenced by a horse's stance. Vet Radiol Ultrasound 2017; 58(1):10–7.

18. Eliashar E. An evidence-based assessment of the biomechanical effects of the common shoeing and farriery techniques. Vet Clin North Am 2007;23:425–42.

19. Redden R. Radiographic imaging of the equine foot. Vet Clin North Am 2003;19: 443–62.

20. Bushe T, Turner T, Poulos P, et al. The effect of hoof angle on coffin, pastern and fetlock joint angles, in Proceedings. Am Assoc Equine Pract 1988;33:729–38.

21. Back W, Schamhardt HC, Hartman W, et al. Kinematic differences between the distal portions of the forelimbs and hind limbs of horses at the trot. Am J Vet Res 1995;56:1552–8.

22. Redden RF. A technique for performing digital venography in the standing horse. Equine Vet Educ 2001;3(3):172–8.

23. Redden R. Hoof capsule distortions: Understanding the mechanisms as a basis for rational management. Vet Clin North Am 2003;19:443–62.

24. Balch OK. The effects of change in hoof angle, mediolateral balance, and toe length on kinetic and temporal parameters of horse walking, trotting and cantering on a high-speed treadmill (ph thesis). Pullman (WA): Washington State University; 1993. p. 21–30.

25. Dyhre-Poulsen P, Smedegaard HH, Roed J, et al. Equine hoof function investigated by pressure transducers inside the hoof and accelerometers mounted on the first phalanx. Equine Vet J 1994;26:362–6.

26. Rooney JR. The lame horse: causes, symptoms, and treat- ment. Chatsworth, CA: Wilshire Book Co; 1974. p. 117–8.

27. Bowker RM. The anatomy of the ungula cartilage and digital cushion. 12th Annual Bluegrass Laminitis Symposium 75-88. 1998.

28. Peel J, Peel M, Davies H. The Effect of gallop training on hoof angle in the thoroughbred racehorses. Equine Vet Supplementary 2006;36:43.

Endocrinopathic Laminitis

Nora S. Grenager, VMD

KEYWORDS

- Laminitis • Insulin dysregulation • Insulin resistance • Metabolic syndrome
- Endocrinopathy • Pituitary pars intermedia dysfunction

KEY POINTS

- Endocrinopathic laminitis, due primarily to hyperinsulinemia, is a relatively non-inflammatory pathophysiology of laminitis.
- Insulin likely acts via insulin-like growth factor receptor-1 in the lamina to set off pathways that lead to lamellar proliferation, stretching, and failure of the suspensory apparatus of the distal phalanx.
- Endocrinopathic laminitis is preventable in many circumstances, especially with early recognition of risk factors or clinical signs.
- Annual hoof evaluation plus screening all geriatric horses for pituitary pars intermedia dysfunction and insulin dysregulation (ID), and younger horses for ID, will allow prevention or early recognition.

INTRODUCTION

In recent years, 3 main causes for laminitis have been elucidated: endocrinopathic (including pasture-associated; also called "hyperinsulinemic-associated laminitis"), systemic inflammatory response syndrome (SIRS) -associated, and support limb (contralateral limb); a fourth, less common, cause is trauma. Although there are overlaps and similarities among these conditions, endocrinopathic laminitis (EL) has critical distinctions from the others in its pathophysiology, presentation, and treatment. It is helpful to recognize these differences to maximize the potential to prevent, diagnose, and treat this devastating condition.

BACKGROUND
Relationship Between Endocrinopathic Laminitis, Insulin Dysregulation, and Pituitary Pars Intermedia Dysfunction

Insulin dysregulation (ID) is defined as any combination of resting hyperinsulinemia, abnormal oral or intravenous (IV) carbohydrate test response, or tissue insulin resistance (IR) (**Table 1**). Likely the key pathophysiologic factor of EL, ID has repeatedly been shown to be associated with an increased risk of laminitis.[1] Equine metabolic syndrome (EMS) is defined as a syndrome of ID, increased risk of EL, and regional or generalized

Steinbeck Peninsula Equine Clinics, 100 Ansel Lane, Menlo Park, CA 94028, USA
E-mail address: ngrenagervmd@gmail.com

Vet Clin Equine 37 (2021) 619–638
https://doi.org/10.1016/j.cveq.2021.08.001
0749-0739/21/© 2021 Elsevier Inc. All rights reserved.

Table 1
Definitions surrounding insulin dynamics in horses

Condition	Definition	Laboratory Findings
Insulin dysregulation	Broad term for abnormal insulin dynamics in the body	≥ 1 of insulin resistance, tissue insulin resistance, or postprandial hyperinsulinemia
Postprandial hyperinsulinemia	Body overreacts to glucose, increasing insulin secretion from pancreatic β cells to maintain normoglycemia; insulin returns to normal range between meals	Insulin > reference range at 60 and/or 90 min after meal or oral sugar/glucose
Insulin resistance (hyperinsulinemia)	Pancreatic β-cell secretion increases to maintain normal blood glucose levels in the face of decreased cellular insulin sensitivity	Serum insulin is above reference range at all time points (fasting, fed); positive IV insulin tolerance test

adiposity. One-third to two-thirds of equids with pituitary pars intermedia dysfunction (PPID) have documented ID.[2,3] The 2 most common equine endocrinopathies, PPID and EMS, are both associated with EL, likely due, at least in part, to the ID, abnormal adiposity, and probable cortisol dysregulation seen with these conditions.

Relationship Between Pituitary Pars Intermedia Dysfunction and Insulin Dysregulation

It remains to be determined whether PPID and ID are independent comorbidities or related conditions (ie, PPID causes ID or vice versa). It may be coincidental that equids with ID develop PPID as they age, because both conditions are common. Alternatively, PPID may cause or exacerbate ID, or there may be an underlying genetic predisposition to both conditions. Insulin dysregulation (ID) with PPID could be due to the increased pro-opiomelanocortin (POMC)-derived peptides of PPID acting as insulin secretagogues in pancreatic beta cells and/or obesity/PPID/aging may decrease hepatic insulin clearance.[3] In addition, the proinflammatory profile and chronic hyperglycemia of adiposity may drive ID. Finally, there are documented age-related declines in insulin sensitivity in horses like what is seen in other species.[3]

There may be aspects of PPID aside from ID that cause laminitis, although the histopathology of naturally occurring laminitis associated with PPID is like that of laminitis induced by hyperinsulinemia in research studies. Furthermore, suggesting that ID is key in the development of EL in horses with PPID, laminar histopathologic findings are often normal in PPID-positive horses that have normal resting insulin.[4] However, although 1 group found that horses with PPID and hyperinsulinemia develop laminitis but those with normal insulin rarely develop laminitis,[4] another found laminitis in all PPID horses in their study, just of decreased severity in the normoinsulinemic group.[3] Unfortunately, dynamic insulin testing was not performed in the latter study, so it is possible that ID was missed in some cases.

Additional Pathways to Endocrinopathic Laminitis

In addition to EMS and PPID, EL can be associated with exogenous corticosteroid administration or access to lush pasture in horses with underlying, although frequently previously undiagnosed, ID.

Many studies have found that administering steroids to horses without known risk factors (**Table 2**) does not induce laminitis.[5–7] The risk of EL associated with steroids depends on the horse's underlying risk factors; concurrent illness(es); and the type, dose, route, and duration of administration. Potter and colleagues[8] recently reported an odds ratio of 18.23 for developing laminitis after corticosteroid administration in horses with known ID, PPID, or previous laminitis.[5] Intra-articular or local (eg, ophthalmic, dermal, inhaled) therapy carries a lower risk of inducing or exacerbating ID than intravenous (IV) or intramuscular (IM) administration because less is absorbed systemically. Recent work by Haseler and colleagues[6] compared 966 client-owned horses treated or not treated with intra-articular triamcinolone and found no difference in the incidence of laminitis in the 4 months following treatment. However, the clinicians may have accounted for the risk factors for EL when selecting cases for therapy because they were client-owned horses. By now it is accepted that the administration of steroids, such as triamcinolone or dexamethasone, to horses with risk factors can be the "domino" to set off an episode of clinical laminitis.

Pasture-associated laminitis is likely associated with ID set off by high concentrations of nonstructural carbohydrates (NSC) found in some pastures.[9] This has been demonstrated in many studies, including a documented increased incidence of EL in spring in the northern hemisphere, presumably associated with pasture type and access at that time of year.[10]

There is also almost certainly a genetic risk for EMS—ponies, and Spanish breeds, gaited breeds, Morgans, miniature horses, and Arabians are overrepresented.[11] However, a review of 199 cases of EL and pasture-associated laminitis by Coleman and colleagues[10] found no association between breed and EL incidence.

CHARACTERIZATION OF ENDOCRINOPATHIC LAMINITIS

The common feature among the primary laminitis causes remains failure of the suspensory apparatus of the distal phalanx. This is associated with stretching, crushing, and distortion of the local dermal/epidermal tissues and bone, leading to abnormal hoof growth and secondary pathologic conditions (eg, foot abscesses, osteopenia, and [micro-] fractures of the distal phalanx).[12] We histologically see this common epidermal lamellar pathologic condition at both acute and chronic stages of laminitis,[12,13] and it can even be grossly visible with chronic laminitis (eg, lamellar wedge lesions, divergent growth rings).[14] The lesions, location, and degree of local inflammation vary depending on the cause, rapidity of onset, and predisposing biomechanics of the foot.[15]

The primary lesion with EL is stretching, elongation, and proliferation of the laminae. The euglycemic-hyperinsulinemic clamp (EHC) causes elongation of secondary

Table 2		
Risk factors for endocrinopathic laminitis		
Historical Findings	**Physical Examination Findings**	**Farrier Findings**
PPID—documented or suspected	Adiposity—regional or generalized	Stretched white line
ID—documented	Additional clinical signs of PPID (eg, hypertrichosis)	Bruised sole
Sore after trimming	Divergent hoof growth/rings	Recurrent hoof abscesses
Sore after turnout onto pasture	Radiographic evidence of laminar inflammation	

epidermal lamellae (SEL) and increased apoptosis in the developmental phase.[16,17] The primary histopathologic findings of EL include widening and lengthening of primary epidermal lamellae (PEL), tapering and fusion of PEL and SEL, mitotic figures in the SEL; apoptotic cells; and proliferation, keratinization, and separation of the epidermis from the underlying dermis.[4]

Naturally occurring chronic cases of EL have tapered and lengthened SEL, irregular SEL fusion and replacement with keratinized tissue, epithelial islands, and increased apoptotic cells.[13]

Endocrinopathic Laminitis Is Primarily Non-inflammatory

The primary lesion with SIRS-associated laminitis is injury to the basement membrane (BM) resulting in significant local inflammation and separation of the epidermal and dermal lamellae.[13] There is less widespread inflammation and epidermal apoptosis in the developmental stages of EL,[13] and instead elongation and apoptosis of SEL are seen, largely in the absence of injury to the BM with relatively minimal inflammation.[16] Karikoski and colleagues[13] found that 50% to 70% of the SEL were markedly tapered and elongated in chronic EL compared with controls (5%–10%), especially in abaxial regions of hoof, where there was also SEL fusion, presence of abnormal keratinized tissue, and numerous apoptotic cells.

PREVALENCE

It has been repeatedly found that EL is the most common type of laminitis, causing up to 90% of clinical laminitis cases.[1] Up to 34% of horses will be affected with laminitis in their lifetime.[18] This is likely associated with the fact that 21% to 30% of equids older than 15 years of age are diagnosed with PPID,[2,3] and 30% of those (independent of insulin status) develops laminitis.[19]

The lifestyle of our modern-day equine population in developed countries where horses are not used for household work likely contributes to this prevalence of EL. In the United States, 19% of horses are clinically obese, while 32% are overweight.[20] Although reportedly 18% to 27% of horses are hyperinsulinemic (in the United States and Australia, respectively), statistics regarding prevalence of ID or EMS in the horse population are lacking.[21,22]

In addition, ID (transient or chronic) can be a compounding issue in many horses suffering from SIRS-associated laminitis. Hospitalized or stressed horses that develop laminitis often have ID, exacerbating (or, this author would suggest, possibly predisposing to) what has historically been considered SIRS-associated laminitis. Lipopolysaccharide infusion results in peripheral tissue IR—more significant in horses with EMS but also occurring in horses with normal baseline insulin regulation—and horses with naturally occurring SIRS undergo transient pancreatic dysfunction, perhaps leading to ID.[23,24]

ASSESSMENT, EVALUATION, AND DIAGNOSIS

Clinical laminitis of any cause has the hallmark feature of foot pain, but often EL is more insidious and milder in nature than, in particular, SIRS-associated laminitis.[15] This is further supported by the finding that histopathologic evidence of laminitis occurs before clinical onset of EL,[13,15] and often there is radiographic or gross evidence of previous bouts of laminar inflammation that went clinically unnoticed.

The presentation of horses with EL is more variable compared with other types of laminitis. The 2 main situations in which practitioners evaluate horses with EL include chronic/subclinical cases unnoticed by owners and active cases (acute or acute-on-chronic/flareups). In either situation, there may have been multiple bouts of laminar inflammation preceding the evaluation.

Looking for Chronic Cases Unnoticed by Owners

Hoof evaluation

Unfortunately, owners are not particularly astute at noticing mild bouts of laminar inflammation, and horses with ID can have repeated mild episodes that have gone undetected. Tadros and colleagues[3] reviewed the records of 38 client-owned PPID-positive horses and ponies and noted resting serum insulin, any history of laminitis, and lateral foot radiographic findings. They used this information to categorize the horses as laminitic (mild/moderate/severe) or normal. Radiographs revealed evidence of laminitis in 76% of cases, whereas owners reported a previous laminitis episode in just 37%. Resting insulin levels were higher in those with more significant radiographic changes, and owners were more likely to have noted laminitis with increasing severity of hyperinsulinemia. Last, owners reported laminitis more often in hyperinsulinemic horses compared with those with normal resting insulin. However, no dynamic testing was performed, so some horses probably had undocumented ID.[3]

Close evaluation of the hoof can often reveal abnormal hoof growth or irregularities of the white line (**Fig. 1**). It takes 3 months for divergent growth rings (ie, wider at heels) to be visible after an episode of laminar inflammation.[13] Owners may note (upon questioning) soreness after shoeing/trimming or have received input from the farrier that there was bruising or stretching of the white line (**Fig. 2**). These findings have been associated with increased risk of laminitis,[25] and—because they may occur without clinical lameness—can be a warning sign that allows us to "right the ship."[13]

Response to hoof testers should be evaluated as a baseline. In most cases, radiographs are indicated in these horses to determine what, if any, degree of radiographically evident laminar damage has occurred and to serve as a baseline for follow-up evaluation. Miniature horses and ponies are particularly prone to having rather significant radiographic findings (**Fig. 3**) in the face of no known episodes of laminitis (according to the owner).

Endocrine testing

It is critical to evaluate a horse's endocrine status at this stage in order to have the biggest impact on mitigating the risk of a "full-blown" (ie, severe) laminitic episode.

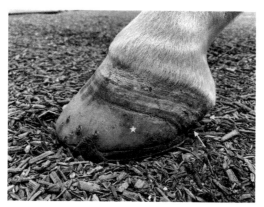

Fig. 1. Divergent hoof growth (*arrows*) and bruising (*star*) consistent with previous episodes of laminitis.

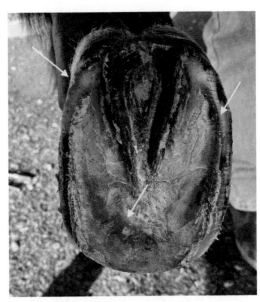

Fig. 2. Bruising of the solar surface of the foot (*arrows*).

At a minimum, measure resting insulin in all horses suspect for ID along with adreno-corticotropic hormone (ACTH) in suspicious horses older than 10 years of age. Evaluate suspect horses that are not positive on these screening first-line tests with dynamic testing (oral sugar test [OST] or insulin tolerance test for ID and thyrotropin-releasing hormone [TRH] stimulation test for PPID).[19] It has been shown

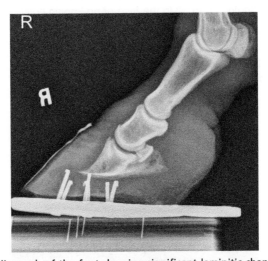

Fig. 3. Lateral radiograph of the foot showing significant laminitic changes (ie, thickened hoof-lamellar zone, rotation of the distal phalanx with respect to the hoof wall, and remodeling of the dorsodistal tip of the distal phalanx) in a miniature horse with no history of lameness noted by the owner. Note the barium paste on the dorsal hoof wall to highlight the wall and level of the coronary band, and the nails in the block, which are a known distance from each other, used to calibrate the image.

to be safe and accurate to perform the TRH stimulation test immediately before an OST to minimize the number of visits.[26]

Looking at Actively Laminitic Cases

Clinical suspicion should drive initial diagnostics and therapeutics.

Hoof evaluation and physical examination

The evaluation of a foot-sore horse suspect for laminitis should include close inspection of the hooves (as described in the previous section, plus careful palpation of coronary bands to identify any sinking of the distal phalanx), assessment of basic physical examination parameters, and physical evaluation for evidence of underlying endocrinopathy, such as EMS or PPID. A few physical examination findings have been evaluated as risk factors for EL (see **Table 2**) and are quick and easy to do once the clinician is accustomed to assessing them.

Increased adiposity (regional or global) is the most obvious finding, which is both common sense and has been shown to be a risk factor for EL. There is also a negative correlation between height and insulin concentration.[27]

The clinician should perform a body condition score (BCS) using a BCS chart, take photographs of the horse from both sides and multiple angles for future comparison, estimate weight (use the same weight tape each time, as there is considerable variation) or weigh the horse, and consider using the cresty neck score (CNS). Fitzgerald and colleagues[28] showed that ponies with a CNS of ≥ 3 were 5 times more likely to have ID than those without, and that CNS was better able to predict ID than was BCS.

The clinician should also be accustomed to looking for additional specific clinical signs of PPID because of the high prevalence of EL in horses with PPID—in particular, hypertrichosis, delayed shedding, or the presence of long guard hairs.

Assessment of pain and Obel scoring

Do not force an acutely laminitic horse to move solely to facilitate a "lameness" examination or to assign an Obel grade. Horses with EL do not always show the same degree of pain, hoof tester response (almost 50% have no response!), or radiographic changes as with other types of laminitis.[15,29]

The original Obel grading scale for laminitis was developed in 1948 using sepsis-associated cases of laminitis. Meier and colleagues[15] found that Obel grading and routine pain scoring are not always correlative to pain level or severity of laminitis in horses with EL. They proposed amending the Obel grading system to reflect what is clinically found with EL, incorporating digital pulses, different stances, and other ways to evaluate movement while removing hoof tester sensitivity as a factor. From this, they developed a 3-step, 5-criteria, 12-point scaled Obel grading system for EL. This new Obel grading system demonstrated excellent interobserver agreement and reproducibility, and substantial repeatability.[15] Whether the clinician uses the system routinely, familiarity with it helps guide more repeatable and objective assessment of these cases.

Radiographs

Radiographic evaluation for EL can be similar to that used in other types of laminitis. It is helpful to mark the coronary band on the lateral views with a radiopaque marker (see **Fig. 3**). It is particularly useful to calibrate the images for more accurate measurements (ie, placing a radiopaque marker of known length into the block or on the hoof wall or sole; see **Fig. 3**; **Fig. 4**).

Any of the hallmark radiographic changes of laminitis may be seen, but we see stretching or thickening of the hoof-lamellar zone (see **Fig. 4**) or indications of previous

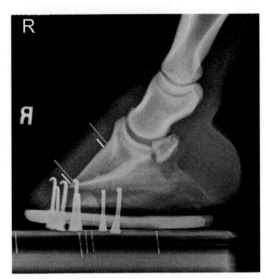

Fig. 4. Lateral radiograph of a foot showing stretching of the distal hoof-lamellar zone (*yellow lines*) in the absence of significant rotation of the distal phalanx with respect to the hoof wall (*orange lines*). Note the nails in the block, which are a known distance from each other, used to calibrate the image.

bouts of laminitis (see **Fig. 3**) with EL more often than might be noted with other types of acute laminitis. Additional common radiographic findings with laminitis in general include rotation or sinking of the distal phalanx with respect to the hoof wall, gas lucencies in the hoof wall, decreased sole depth, remodeling or osteopenia of the dorsodistal tip of the distal phalanx ("ski-tip" appearance), and the presence of a lamellar wedge.[30]

Hormone profiles

It is challenging to accurately assess resting insulin and ACTH in acutely laminitic horses because both values can be increased by stress and pain. For example, even trailering a horse for just 40 minutes increases basal ACTH for at least 30 minutes.[31] Some clinicians advocate that it is worth testing insulin when examining a horse with acute laminitis if there is poor likelihood of follow-up or client compliance. This author typically initially treats endocrinopathies based on clinical suspicion (eg, an overweight horse with laminitis will be started on a course of thyroxine; a hirsute horse with laminitis will be started on pergolide) and typically does not measure ACTH and insulin during acute episodes but prefers to wait until pain has subsided and levels are likely to be more representative of the horse's underlying endocrine state.

CURRENT RESEARCH REGARDING ENDOCRINOPATHIC LAMINITIS

Broadly, insulin-mediated laminitis is characterized by proliferation and stretching of lamellar cells leading to loss of lamellar integrity, with minimal inflammation and possible alterations in local blood flow and metabolism. The current prevailing theory is that hyperinsulinemia causes inappropriate stimulation of insulin-like growth factor-1 receptor (IGF-1R) on laminar epidermal cells, setting off a cascade of downstream events resulting in the laminar changes seen with EL.

Brief Summary of Historical Research

Hyperinsulinemia can directly cause laminitis, as first shown by 2 induction models from 2008 and 2012.[16,32] First, 5 healthy ponies with no known history of laminitis or IR developed Obel grade 2 laminitis after 72 hours of an EHC, resulting in a mean insulin serum level of 1036 microunits per milliliter in the absence of signs of systemic illness.[32] Next, the EHC induced histopathologic laminitis in 4 horses over 48 hours, demonstrating a threshold for insulin toxicity of around 200 microunits per milliliter.[16] It has also been shown that explant lamellae incubated in insulin fail at lower stress and load compared with those incubated in a plain medium.[33] Although these induction models used levels of hyperinsulinemia not physiologically seen in most cases, they demonstrated that insulin can directly cause laminitis in horses.

The magnitude of hyperinsulinemia required to cause clinical EL surely must vary, depending on the degree of preexisting laminar pathologic condition, chronicity, hoof biomechanics, and the individual horse's susceptibility.

Differences in Laminar Inflammation with Endocrinopathic Laminitis

The inflammation that occurs with SIRS-associated laminitis has been well-described at various stages of the carbohydrate overload model of laminitis, with significant lamellar neutrophilic accumulation and activity (see Britta Leise and Lee Ann Fugler's article, "Laminitis Updates: Sepsis/SIRS Associated Laminitis," in this issue). In contrast, several studies have reported minimal evidence of inflammation with both acute and chronic EL.[4,13] In a study by Watts and colleagues,[34] horses underwent EHC or saline infusion for 48 hours or until the onset of Obel grade 1 laminitis and then were humanely euthanized. They measured key cytokines and inflammatory mediators in the digital lamellar tissues using polymerase chain reaction, immunoblotting, and immunohistochemistry. A lack of notable emigration of leukocytes into the lamellar tissue with induced EL implies there is not much "classic inflammation" with EL, despite finding that there were some changes in local cytokine/inflammatory mediator profiles. Those investigators suggest that the lamellar inflammatory signaling they identified may indicate, or be associated with, crosstalk between metabolic regulatory signaling and inflammatory pathways secondary to changes in intracellular concentrations of energetic metabolites rather than be a primary inflammatory event.[34]

Insulin and Insulin-Like Growth Factor-1 Receptor

The actions of insulin and insulin-like growth factor-1 (IGF-1) stimulate lamellar cellular proliferation.[35] Insulin can bind to insulin receptors, IGF-1R, or a hybrid of these.[36] Interestingly, insulin receptors are scarce in lamellar tissue so insulin is unlikely to be mediating its effects directly through them.[37] Furthermore, research has shown that obesity and high-NSC diets lower the types of insulin receptors in a variety of tissues (lamellar, tail head adipose, and liver).[36]

One of the best-supported theories is that insulin stimulates IGF-1R, which then works through several signaling pathways to increase mitosis of lamellar cells, with subsequent stretching and failure. This big-picture theory is complicated by the fact that it apparently requires a very high concentration of insulin that would rarely be seen in vivo. To further confuse matters, it appears insulin does not have much affinity for IGF-1R, and it has been shown that high concentrations of insulin in lamellar tissue causes increased dephosphorylated (ie, inactive) IGF-1R.[37,38] Although it has thus been proposed that insulin instead works through insulin/IGF-1R hybrid receptors, these have not yet been identified in lamellar tissue.[38]

Nevertheless, numerous studies have demonstrated that insulin and IGF-1R play pivotal roles in EL, whether directly or indirectly. Rahnama and colleagues[35] pretreated half the limbs of 13 horses with anti-IGF-1R antibody and then used the EHC to induce laminitis. This led to decreased effects of insulin and IGF-1 (ie, decreased lamellar cellular proliferation) in pretreated limbs, suggesting that insulin acted via IGF-1R. Not all of the effects of insulin were attenuated by the antibody; yet, compared with the positive-control group, horses treated with the antibody had milder histologic changes and less sinking of the distal phalanx, along with significantly decreased elongation at the tips of the SEL.[35] This role of IGF-1R was further demonstrated in another study in which insulin-stimulated cellular proliferation in isolated lamellar cells in vitro was blocked using a selective antihuman IGF-1R monoclonal antibody.[39]

The downstream signaling events following IGF-1R activation are similar across mammalian species. Two main signaling pathways regulated by IGF-1R include Ras/Raf/ERK 1/2 (MAPK) and PI3K/Akt, the former of which regulates cellular proliferation, differentiation, and motility and the latter of which increases cellular proliferation and dysregulation of cellular adhesion.[40] Together these activate mammalian target of rapamycin complex-1 (mTORC1) and RPS6, leading to disruption of cytoskeletal organization, cellular proliferation/differentiation, hemidesmosome dysadhesion, and cellular proliferation, which may disturb lamellar cellular morphology and lead to the lamellar stretching seen with EL.[40] Lane and colleagues[40] looked at these mTORC1/RPS6 protein signaling pathways in lean and obese ponies on low- or high-NSC diets and Standardbreds undergoing EHC and found increased levels in obese ponies on high-NSC diets and Standardbreds undergoing the EHC to induce EL.

Interestingly, IGF-1R plays a pivotal role in cancers as well, activation of which leads to increased mitotic rate, cytoskeletal dysregulation, and decreased adherence of epithelial cells to the BM (mammalian skin and equine hoof wall have a similar BM, basal epithelial layer, dermis, and adhesion complexes).[40] This may be relevant or similar to what is happening in lamellar tissues with EL. These further downstream proteins (mTORC1 and RPS6) appear to be activated during hyperinsulinemia and are culprits for the epithelial dysplasia associated with some cancers. It has been shown that mTORC1 likely activates RPS6, which then disrupts cytoskeletal regulation, affecting lamellar epithelial morphology.[40]

Vascular Dysfunction

Stokes and colleagues[41] induced laminitis in 8 standardbreds via 48 hours of EHC and measured glucose, lactate, and pyruvate (indicators of metabolism and perfusion) in lamellar tissues using tissue microdialysis. They found no effect of hyperinsulinemia on lamellar energy metabolism or perfusion, nor evidence of ischemia, hypoperfusion, or energy stress during the developmental phase. However, the investigators suggest that these factors could play a bigger role in more chronic laminitis, which was not evaluated in this work.[41]

It has been suggested that EL may be, at least in part, caused by vascular dysfunction similar to the peripheral neuropathy seen in humans with metabolic syndrome. Humans with endocrine disease have systemic vascular dysfunction, especially endothelial dysfunction, and subsequent vasodilation. In humans, hyperinsulinemia causes stimulation of the MAPK pathway with production of endothelin-1 and reactive oxygen species. This has also been shown in ex vivo models of equine vessels incubated with high concentrations of insulin.[42] Not surprisingly, however, this stimulation of MAPK is not a clear-cut pathway, as it was found to be downregulated in the lamellar tissues of horses with EL induced via the EHC clamp.[34]

Morgan and colleagues[42] evaluated the response of facial and laminar vessels to vasoconstrictors and vasodilators in horses with EL and non-EL controls. They identified significant vascular dysfunction in both laminar vessels and facial skin arteries in horses with EL (worse in laminar veins compared with others evaluated), demonstrated as blunting of endothelium-dependent vasodilation. Also, the laminar vessels in horses with EL were more responsive to vasoconstrictors. The effect seen in facial arteries suggests that this endothelial dysfunction could be associated with underlying endocrinopathy and not specific to local changes in the hoof. They proposed that this poor venous vasodilation plus excessive arterial vasoconstriction in hooves with EL is a clue that increased capillary pressure and hypoxia of the laminar tissue may drive the changes seen with EL.[42]

Other Mechanisms

Adipose tissue is metabolically active with a proinflammatory phenotype, demonstrating increased gene expression and secretion of proinflammatory cytokines. These proinflammatory activities may be associated with ID seen in equids with regional or global adiposity and, thus, with the development of laminitis. However, a direct link between inflammatory adipokines and laminitis has not been demonstrated.[43]

Horses with ID may also have disordered nutrient sensing and metabolism within the digital lamellae, predisposing or contributing to laminitis. Two very important nutrient substrate flux signaling pathways in the lamellae include the previously mentioned mTORC1 (increases with more glucose/nutrients) and adenosine 50-monophosphate-activated protein kinase (AMPK; increases when under energetic stress).[34] These pathways work together with inflammatory pathways to help regulate inflammatory responses; so, their malfunction may lead to local inflammation and lamellar disturbance.

Leptin is another area of interest because many horses with EMS have hyperleptinemia. Work by Watts and colleagues[34] suggests that leptin receptors in keratinocytes are activated during ID, causing activation of signal transducer and activator of transcription (STAT) proteins: STAT-1 and -3. Of note, an increase of STAT-1 has been identified with sepsis-associated laminitis. In contrast, Burns and colleagues[44] found there was downregulation of expression of leptin and its receptor in an EHC EL induction protocol.

Campolo and colleagues[45] evaluated proteins that were altered in the lamellar tissue of a hyperinsulinemic group of standardbreds (induced via EHC) as compared with controls. Proteins that were increased included those involved in coagulation and complement cascades, platelet activity, and ribosomal function, whereas proteins that were decreased were involved in focal adhesions, spliceosomes, and cell-cell matrices. This suggests that hyperinsulinemia induced some microvascular damage, complement activation, and ribosomal dysfunction in the lamellae. A similar effect was not seen when they evaluated the cardiac tissue of these horses for similar indicators, suggesting that it was unique to the lamellae, or at least not global. They identified an increase in inflammatory markers and heat shock protein-90 (HSP90) during insulin-induced laminitis, but also a decrease of significant cell-cell matrix and focal adhesion proteins. It has been shown that HSP90 is higher in type 2 human diabetics, and treating with an HSP90 inhibitor improves kidney function and treats atherosclerosis; this may be indicative of its effects in the lamellar tissues.[45]

Cassimeris and colleagues[14] investigated whether chronic overstimulation of pro-growth and anabolic pathways in the lamellar tissue leads to stress on the endoplasmic reticulum (ER).[14] They evaluated protein markers of ER stress from the lamellar tissue of horses with naturally occurring EL. They found evidence that this stress does occur and results in the unfolded protein response (which is known to cause loss of cellular function in human diabetics), especially in the thoracic limbs. Thoracic limbs may be more susceptible to ER stress because of both increased energy demand and decreased nutrient delivery associated with limb-loading differences. Laminitis is more common in thoracic than pelvic limbs because the thoracic limbs carry 60% of a horse's body weight. This increased body weight on the front hooves likely impacts the mechanics of digital suspension and lamellar perfusion, subsequently affecting cellular energy balance and homeostatic capabilities.[46,47] Furthermore, ER stress may activate mTORC1, which as described previously can set off a cascade of lamellar events leading to EL.[14]

DISCUSSION OF CLINICAL RELEVANCE OF CURRENT RESEARCH

Some of the specific cytokines, proteins, and pathways discussed may provide more specific targets of future therapeutics, but at this time, clinically applicable inhibitors of IGF-1R, mTORC1, AMPK, RSP6, MAPK, PI3K, STAT proteins, and HSP90 are either not available or not yet evaluated in veterinary medicine. For example, rapamycin is a therapeutic used to diminish malignancy and tumor growth in human epithelial cancers because of its ability to block mTORC1, which could prevent some of the downstream lamellar signaling events leading to EL. However, it requires further evaluation in equids and clinically would likely need to be used in conjunction with other therapies because it has shown some toxicity in human trials.[40]

Overall, this body of work from the last decade suggests that therapies directed at improving perfusion during the developmental phase of EL would not be appropriate,[41] inhibitors of IGF-1R and mTORC1/ER stress pathways may be indicated, and that it is critical to decrease the presence and activity of adipose tissue to address ID. This recent work brings to light some promising novel therapeutic options that merit further investigation in the equine population.

THERAPEUTIC APPROACH

There are 3 prongs of treatment for laminitis of any cause: address the underlying cause when known (ID $\pm$ PPID for EL), administer anti-inflammatories/analgesics, and provide biomechanically appropriate hoof support.

Decrease Insulin

Pharmaceuticals

Thyroxine and metformin are the primary pharmaceutical interventions clinically available to improve insulin sensitivity in horses. Sodium-glucose co-transporter 2 (SGLT2) inhibitors (eg, velagliflozin) are currently costly and thus only applicable in specific situations.

In 2008, Frank and colleagues[48] first showed that long-term oral administration of levothyroxine was associated with weight loss and increased insulin sensitivity in 6 adult euthyroid horses. In 2010, this was followed by a study that showed that insulin sensitivity decreased with hospitalization and endotoxemia; this was aggravated by dexamethasone and improved by thyroxine administration.[49] It is now widely accepted that thyroxine improves insulin sensitivity, and its use is indicated in acutely laminitic obese patients or obese patients with ID that do not respond to diet and exercise. Based on these data, this author also uses thyroxine to help mitigate anticipated ID when steroid administration is necessary in a horse with risk factors for EL.

Metformin has gained popularity for short-term use to safely reduce glycemic and insulinemic responses in horses that remain hyperinsulinemic despite diet and management changes.[50,51] Metformin has poor bioavailability in horses with minimal absorption.[52] However, it has been shown in humans, and suggested in equids, to work at the level of the enterocytes to decrease glucose absorption because it does reduce insulin concentrations in treated horses.[51] Metformin is thus most efficacious when administered orally 30 minutes before feeding.

The SGLT2 inhibitors are gaining in popularity for clients with the financial resources to pay for them. These medications reduce renal glucose reabsorption and promote glucosuria, thus decreasing blood glucose and, subsequently, insulin concentrations. Meier and colleagues[53] looked at effects of velagliflozin in ponies with IR fed high-NSC diets. The maximum insulin in the treated group was 45% lower than that in the controls. The diet induced Obel grade 1 or 2 laminitis in 14 of 37 controls (38%), but no velagliflozin-treated pony developed laminitis. The treatment did not cause any noted ill effects or hypoglycemia in this study.[53] However, these drugs reportedly cause hyperlipemia and therefore should not be used in hypertriglyceridemic equids.[19]

Pioglitazone is a thiazolidinedione that decreases OST response and adiponectin levels in horses with EMS.[54]

Exercise

Exercise (even just 30 minutes a day, 5 days a week, including brisk trotting) is an inexpensive method to help improve insulin sensitivity, provided the horse's feet are stable enough to tolerate it.[55,56] Unfortunately, actively laminitic horses or those recovering from recent flareups cannot undergo enough exercise to improve insulin sensitivity, even if they are walking a bit of their own accord around their enclosure. Furthermore, client compliance can be difficult for a variety of reasons: the clients' schedules, clients' health issues, or the horse's management situation.

Exercise needs to occur as close to daily as possible to affect insulin sensitivity. Powell and colleagues[57] found that just 30 minutes of trotting exercise each day for 7 days improved insulin sensitivity by 60% in obese mares (and by 48% in lean mares) for 24 hours after exercise but not for much longer.

Treat pituitary pars intermedia dysfunction

Horses diagnosed with, or highly suspect for, PPID should be treated with a Food and Drug Administration–approved pergolide product in addition to the other management and therapeutic strategies discussed here. Additional management strategies and therapeutics for PPID are beyond the scope of this article.

Diet

Because most horses with EL have ID and/or obesity, most of the dietary recommendations focus on improving insulin sensitivity and promoting weight loss (**Box 1**). The more uncommon lean horses with EL and ID have very different dietary needs. Close attention to diet and a rigid schedule of follow-ups are critical.

Numerous other dietary supplements (eg, chromium, magnesium, cinnamon, turmeric, resveratrol, omega fatty acids, silymarin) have been suggested to help with ID and EL (often extrapolated from human medicine). None have strong research to support their use at this time in equids; however, veterinarians may recommend a specific product based on their experiences.

Appropriate Biomechanics for Hoof Support

Please see Raul Bras and Scott Morrison's article, "Mechanical Principles of the Equine Foot," in this issue.

Box 1
Overview of dietary recommendations for horses with insulin dysregulation[19]

Plan for *obese horse* with insulin dysregulation:
- Estimate the horse's current body weight (BW) and BCS (use the same weight tape each time for consistency); it is helpful to take baseline photographs from multiple angles
- Determine the horse's target BW and BCS
- Weigh the horse's forage and grain intake; also ask about treats (they really add up and owners often forget about them)
- Stop all pasture access and any additional pellets/grains
- If the horse is being fed greater than 2.5% BW per day in forage, reduce to 2% of current BW; if the horse is being fed less than 2.5% BW per day in forage, reduce to 1.5% of current BW
- Suggest a slow-feeder net or bin to minimize boredom and mitigate the risk of developing gastric ulcer syndrome
- Reassess horse's weight (tape and BCS) in 30 days (compare to photographs from day 1 if needed)
- If weight loss has not been achieved, can decrease forage to 1.2% of current BW
- Use hays that have been tested and are less than 10% NSC; in cases in which this is not possible (eg, large boarding facilities), the owner can soak the hay for 60 minutes in cold water to decrease water-soluble carbohydrates
- Supplement with a low-NSC ration balancer to meet any additional nutritional (vitamin, mineral, protein) needs; this is especially important if the hay is being soaked

Amended plan for *lean horse* with insulin dysregulation:
- Do not reduce or restrict total forage intake
- Use low-NSC forage and feeds as discussed above
- Use high-fat supplementation to meet caloric needs

Pasture access:
- Horses with ID should be allowed on pasture only once other risk factors have been mitigated as much as possible
- Unfortunately, large pasture turnout will likely never be appropriate for these cases
- However, once the horse has a normal OST result, slow reintroduction may be possible[17]
- Use of a grazing muzzle may be indicated, although equids can adapt and take in much more grass than expected through the muzzle, and some do not tolerate its use
- When possible, pasture or dry lot are better for horses than a small stall where no exercise occurs

---

Anti-Inflammatory and Analgesic Therapy

To avoid redundancy with Klaus Hopster's article, "Pharmacology of the Equine Foot - Medical Pain Management for Laminitis," in this issue, this section focuses on the types of management typically needed in horses with EL, which is often less severely painful than other types of laminitis.

Nonsteroidal anti-inflammatories

Nonsteroidal anti-inflammatories (NSAIDs) remain the mainstay of anti-inflammatory and analgesic therapy for laminitis. Although there is less inflammation associated with EL compared with other causes, there is still some, and the analgesic effects further warrant their use. Phenylbutazone and flunixin meglumine provide an adequate level of analgesia in many cases, but they are nonselective cyclooxygenase (COX) inhibitors and may cause gastrointestinal ulceration and nephrotoxicosis.

The COX-1–sparing NSAIDs (eg, firocoxib and meloxicam) are gaining popularity because of the decreased (although still real) risk of side effects. Although COX-2 was shown to be upregulated during the developmental stage of laminitis induced by black walnut extract,[58] these more selective NSAIDs unfortunately typically do not provide adequate analgesia for an acutely laminitic patient. However, they may be a better option for treating chronic laminitis because it has been shown that COX-2 is increased in these cases, and the need for analgesia may be decreased.[34,59]

Gabapentin

Gabapentin is an analogue of the inhibitory neurotransmitter gamma-aminobutyric acid that acts as an analgesic and anticonvulsant. It has been recommended for use in horses (some sedation is seen at higher doses) to help prevent the "wind-up" phenomenon associated with laminar pain.

Phosphodiesterase inhibitors

Pentoxifylline acts as an inhibitor of matrix metalloproteinase-9 and -2, improves blood flow by making erythrocytes more deformable, and has anti-inflammatory effects.[60,61] With minimal to no known side effects and several possible benefits, it is often part of the acute therapeutic plan.

Cryotherapy

Please see Daniela Luethy's article "Cryotherapy Techniques – Best Protocols to Support the Foot in Health and Disease," in this issue.

PROGNOSIS

The short-term prognosis for life with EL is typically better than for SIRS-associated laminitis, but there is a high recurrence rate, likely partially (or in this author's opinion, mostly) because of failure to appropriately mitigate the risk factors. Furthermore, weakness of the lamellar interface following an episode of EL (subclinical or clinical) drives the recurrent, chronic nature of the condition. **Box 2** lists typical possible outcomes.

de Laat and colleagues[62] looked at 317 client-owned horses with EL over 2 years and identified a recurrence rate of 34.1% with increased risk associated with increased resting fasting insulin levels. There was a higher risk of laminitis during the study period if the horse had ever had a diagnosis of laminitis; cases with a higher Obel grade were more likely to recur sooner. Notably, normal resting insulin was not useful in prediction of future episodes, likely because it does not consider cases of ID that would be identified with dynamic testing.[62]

One-third of laminitis cases are reportedly humanely euthanized within a year of diagnosis or recur within 2 years.[62,63] Similarly, documented hyperinsulinemia in

---

Box 2
Possible outcomes with acute endocrinopathic laminitis

- Mild acute: No radiographic changes, lameness and clinical signs resolve within days; slow return to work may be possible within weeks, with close attention to risk factors

- Acute-on-chronic/subclinical: Radiographic and/or gross indications of previous laminar inflammation suggest even higher risk of recurrence

- Moderate acute: Mild radiographic changes, horse treated for months, life-long management but possible return to work

- Severe acute: Severe radiographic changes, ends athletic career, possibly necessitates euthanasia

- ■ Perform endocrine testing to guide dietary and management changes ± therapeutics in all of these scenarios.

- ■■ It is critical to warn owner of high risk of recurrence after even 1 clinical episode.

PPID-positive horses is greater than 90% sensitive and specific for nonsurvival within 1 to 2 years, owing to laminitis.[64] These staggering numbers underscore the importance of preventing EL, or early recognition and aggressive treatment when that is not possible.

SUMMARY

EL primarily occurs because of ID mediated through the downstream effects of insulin on IGF-1R in lamellar tissues, although at this time it remains unclear how much insulin binds to IGF-1R, even at supraphysiologic doses. There is likely contributing vascular and metabolic dysfunction within the lamellae, but EL is relatively non-inflammatory. EL is associated with increased lamellar stretching, proliferation, and failure, ultimately causing failure of the suspensory apparatus of the distal phalanx. It can present as an acute episode or, more commonly, there may be multiple episodes of subclinical lamellar damage that go unnoticed by the owner until it reaches a threshold causing clinical laminitis and severe lameness.

Proper education of veterinarians, farriers, and caregivers/clients to pay close attention to mitigating risk factors makes this a preventable cause of laminitis in most instances. Annual hoof evaluation plus screening of all geriatric horses for PPID and ID, and younger horses for ID, can result in a significant decrease in the incidence of this devastating condition.

CLINICS CARE POINTS

- Risk factors for endocrinopathic laminitis include the following: regional or generalized adiposity; abnormal hoof growth; documented insulin dysregulation; documented or suspected pituitary pars intermedia dysfunction; history of sore feet, documented laminitis, stretching or bruising of the white line.
- Evaluate at least annually in horses with any risk factors: weight/body condition score, regional adiposity, hair coat, hoof quality/growth, ± foot radiographs.
- Follow recommendations for screening for horses with risk factors for endocrinopathic laminitis annually, evaluate insulin status plus, in horses over 10 years of age, pituitary pars intermedia dysfunction testing.
- Good routine foot care and a close working relationship with the farrier are essential.
- Use steroids judiciously (or topically/inhaled/local) in horses with risk factors and discuss risk with owner.
- Dietary management is critical; recommend nutritional consultation when appropriate.
- Horses with demonstrated equine metabolic syndrome, pituitary pars intermedia dysfunction, or endocrinopathic laminitis: create a schedule for rechecks to mitigate risk in an ongoing fashion.
- Set client expectations: discuss risk of recurrence with client and work to reduce risk factors.

DISCLOSURE

The author has nothing to disclose.

REFERENCES

1. Karikoski NP, Horn I, McGowan TW, et al. The prevalence of endocrinopathic laminitis among horses presented for laminitis at a first-opinion/referral equine hospital. Domest Anim Endocrinol 2011;41(3):111–7.

2. McGowan TW, Pinchbeck GP, McGowan CM. Prevalence, risk factors and clinical signs predictive for equine pituitary pars intermedia dysfunction in aged horses. Equine Vet J 2013;45(1):74–9.

3. Tadros EM, Fowlie JG, Refsal KR, et al. Association between hyperinsulinaemia and laminitis severity at the time of pituitary pars intermedia dysfunction diagnosis. Equine Vet J 2019;51(1):52–6.

4. Karikoski NP, Patterson-Kane JC, Singer ER, et al. Lamellar pathology in horses with pituitary pars intermedia dysfunction. Equine Vet J 2016;48(4):472–8.

5. Cornelisse CJ, Robinson NE. Glucocorticoid therapy and the risk of equine laminitis. Equine Vet Edu 2013;25(1):39–46.

6. Haseler CJ, Jarvis GE, McGovern KF. Intrasynovial triamcinolone treatment is not associated with incidence of acute laminitis. Equine Vet J 2021;53(5):895–901.

7. Jordan VJ, Ireland JL, Rendle DI. Does oral prednisolone treatment increase the incidence of acute laminitis? Equine Vet J 2017;49(1):19–25.

8. Potter K, Stevens K, Menzies-Gow N. Prevalence of and risk factors for acute laminitis in horses treated with corticosteroids. Vet Rec 2019;185(3):82.

9. Menzies-Gow NJ, Harris PA, Elliott J. Prospective cohort study evaluating risk factors for the development of pasture-associated laminitis in the United Kingdom. Equine Vet J 2017;49(3):300–6.

10. Coleman MC, Belknap JK, Eades SC, et al. Case-control study of risk factors for pasture-and endocrinopathy-associated laminitis in North American horses. J Am Vet Med Assoc 2018;253(4):470–8.

11. Durham AE, Frank N, McGowan CM, et al. ECEIM consensus statement on equine metabolic syndrome. J Vet Intern Med 2019;33:335–49.

12. Engiles JB, Galantino-Homer H, Boston R, et al. Osteopathology in the equine distal phalanx associated with the development and progression of laminitis. J Vet Pathol 2015;52:928–44.

13. Karikoski NP, McGowan CM, Singer ER, et al. Pathology of natural cases of equine endocrinopathic laminitis associated with hyperinsulinemia. Vet Pathol 2015;52(5):945–56.

14. Cassimeris L, Engiles JB, Galantino-Homer H. Detection of endoplasmic reticulum stress and the unfolded protein response in naturally-occurring endocrinopathic equine laminitis. BMC Vet Res 2019;15(1):24.

15. Meier A, de Laat M, Pollitt C, et al. A "modified Obel" method for the severity scoring of (endocrinopathic) equine laminitis. PeerJ 2019;7:e7084.

16. de Laat MA, Sillence MN, McGowan CM, et al. Continuous intravenous infusion of glucose induces endogenous hyperinsulinaemia and lamellar histopathology in Standardbred horses. Vet J 2012;191(3):317–22.

17. Asplin KE, Patterson-Kane JC, Sillence MN, et al. Histopathology of insulin-induced laminitis in ponies. Equine Vet J 2010;42(8):700–6.

18. Wylie CE, Collins SN, Verheyen KLP, et al. Frequency of equine laminitis: a systematic review with quality appraisal of published evidence. Vet J 2011;189(3):248–56.

19. Frank NF, Bailey S, Bertin FR, et al. Recommendations for the diagnosis and treatment of equine metabolic syndrome (EMS) from 2020 Equine Endocrinology Group. Available at: https://sites.tufts.edu/equineendogroup/files/2020/09/200592_EMS_Recommendations_Bro-FINAL.pdf. Accessed August 19, 2020.

20. Thatcher CD, Pleasant RS, Geor RJ, et al. Prevalence of obesity in mature horses: an equine body condition study. J Anim Physiol Anim Nutr 2008;92:222.

21. Pleasant RS, Suagee JK, Thatcher CD, et al. Adiposity, plasma insulin, leptin, lipids, and oxidative stress in mature light breed horses. J Vet Intern Med 2013;27(3):576–82.

22. Morgan RA, McGowan TW, McGowan CM. Prevalence and risk factors for hyperinsulinaemia in ponies in Queensland, Australia. Aust Vet J 2014;92(4):101–6.

23. Tadros EM, Frank N, De Witte FG, et al. Effects of intravenous lipopolysaccharide infusion on glucose and insulin dynamics in horses with equine metabolic syndrome. Am J Vet Res 2013;74:1020–9.

24. Bertin FR, Ruffin-Taylor D, Stewart AJ. Insulin dysregulation in horses with systemic inflammatory response syndrome. J Vet Intern Med 2018;32(4):1420–7.

25. Wylie CE, Collins SN, Verheyen KLP, et al. Risk factors for equine laminitis: a case-control study conducted in veterinary-registered horses and ponies in Great Britain between 2009 and 2011. Vet J 2013 Oct;198(1):57–69.

26. Hodge E, Kowalski A, Torcivia C, et al. Effect of thyrotropin-releasing hormone stimulation testing on the oral sugar test in horses when performed as a combined protocol. J Vet Intern Med 2019;33(5):2272–9.

27. de Laat MA, Sillence MN, Reiche DB. Phenotypic, hormonal, and clinical characteristics of equine endocrinopathic laminitis. J Vet Intern Med 2019;33:1456–63.

28. Fitzgerald DM, Anderson ST, Sillence MN, et al. The cresty neck score is an independent predictor of insulin dysregulation in ponies. PLoS One 2019;14(7): e0220203.

29. Meier AD, de Laat MA, Reiche DB, et al. The oral glucose test predicts laminitis risk in ponies fed a diet high in nonstructural carbohydrates. Domest Anim Endocrinol 2018;63:1–9.

30. Sherlock C, Parks A. Radiographic and radiological assessment of laminitis. Equine Vet Educ 2013;25(10):524–35.

31. Haffner JC. Practical clinical research results to consider when testing for PPID in horses. In AAEP proceedings. 2020. Available at: https://aaep.digitellinc.com/ aaep/sessions/4871/view. Accessed August 31, 2020.

32. Asplin KE, Sillence MN, Pollitt CC, et al. Induction of laminitis by prolonged hyperinsulinaemia in clinically normal ponies. Vet J 2007;174(3):530–5.

33. Sandow C, Fugler LA, Leise B, et al. Ex vivo effects of insulin on the structural integrity of equine digital lamellae. Equine Vet J 2019;51(1):131–5.

34. Watts MR, Hegedus OC, Eades SC, et al. Association of sustained supraphysiologic hyperinsulinemia and inflammatory signaling within the digital lamellae in light-breed horses. J Vet Intern Med 2019;33:1483–92.

35. Rahnama S, Vathsangam N, Spence R, et al. Effects of an anti-IGF-1 receptor monoclonal antibody on laminitis induced by prolonged hyperinsulinaemia in standardbred horses. PLoS One 2020;15(9):e0239261.

36. Kullmann A, Weber PS, Bishop JB, et al. Equine insulin receptor and insulin-like growth factor-1 receptor expression in digital lamellar tissue and insulin target tissues. Equine Vet J 2016;48(5):626–32.

37. Rahnama S, Spence R, Vathsangam N, et al. Effects of insulin on IGF-1 receptors in equine lamellar tissue in vitro. Domest Anim Endocrinol 2021;74:106530.

38. Nanayakkara SN, Rahnama S, Harris PA, et al. Characterization of insulin and IGF-1 receptor binding in equine liver and lamellar tissue: implications for endocrinopathic laminitis. Domest Anim Endocrinol 2019;66:21–6.

39. Baskerville CL, Chockalingham S, Harris PA, et al. The effect of insulin on equine lamellar basal epithelial cells mediated by the insulin-like growth factor-1 receptor. PeerJ 2018;6:e5945.

40. Lane HE, Burns TA, Hegedus OC, et al. Lamellar events related to insulin-like growth factor-1 receptor signalling in two models relevant to endocrinopathic laminitis. Equine Vet J 2017;49(5):643–54.

41. Stokes SM, Bertin FR, Stefanovski D, et al. Lamellar energy metabolism and perfusion in the euglycaemic hyperinsulinaemic clamp model of equine laminitis. Equine Vet J 2020;52(4):577–84.

42. Morgan RA, Keen JA, Walker BR, et al. Vascular dysfunction in horses with endocrinopathic laminitis. PLoS One 2016;11(9):e0163815.

43. Burns TA, Geor RJ, Mudge MC, et al. Proinflammatory cytokine and chemokine gene expression profiles in subcutaneous and visceral adipose tissue depots of insulin-resistant and insulin-sensitive light breed horses. J Vet Intern Med 2010;24(4):932–9.

44. Burns TA, Nijveldt E, Watts M, et al. Systemic and local regulation of leptin in a model of endocrinopathic laminitis. In: 2019 ACVIM Forum Research Abstract Program. J Vet Intern Med 2019;33(5):2375–547.

45. Campolo A, Frantz MW, de Laat MA, et al. Differential proteomic expression of equine cardiac and lamellar tissue during insulin-induced laminitis. Front Vet Sci 2020;7:308.

46. Hood DM, Wagner IP, Taylor DD, et al. Voluntary limb-load distribution in horses with acute and chronic laminitis. Am J Vet Res 2001;62:1393–8.

47. Gardner AK, van Eps AW, Watts MR, et al. A novel model to assess lamellar signaling relevant to preferential weight bearing in the horse. Vet J 2017; 221:62–7.

48. Frank N, Elliott SB, Boston RC. Effects of long-term oral administration of levothyroxine sodium on glucose dynamics in healthy adult horses. Am J Vet Res 2008; 69(1):76–81.

49. Tóth F, Frank N, Geor RJ, et al. Effects of pretreatment with dexamethasone or levothyroxine sodium on endotoxin-induced alterations in glucose and insulin dynamics in horses. Am J Vet Res 2010;71(1):60–8.

50. Durham AE, Rendle DI, Newton JE. The effect of metformin on measurements of insulin sensitivity and beta cell response in 18 horses and ponies with insulin resistance. Equine Vet J 2008;40(5):493–500.

51. Rendle DI, Rutledge F, Hughes KJ, et al. Effects of metformin hydrochloride on blood glucose and insulin responses to oral dextrose in horses. Equine Vet J 2013;45(6):751–4.

52. Tinworth KD, Edwards S, Noble GK, et al. Pharmacokinetics of metformin after enteral administration in insulin-resistant ponies. Am J Vet Res 2010;71(10): 1201–6.

53. Meier A, Reiche D, de Laat M, et al. The sodium-glucose co-transporter 2 inhibitor velagliflozin reduces hyperinsulinemia and prevents laminitis in insulin-dysregulated ponies. PLoS One 2018;13(9):e0203655.

54. Legere RM, Taylor DR, Davis JL, et al. Pharmacodynamic effects of pioglitazone on high molecular weight adiponectin concentrations and insulin response after oral sugar in equids. J Equine Vet Sci 2019;82:102797.

55. Bamford NJ, Potter SJ, Baskerville CL, et al. Influence of dietary restriction and low-intensity exercise on weight loss and insulin sensitivity in obese equids. J Vet Intern Med 2019;33(1):280–6.

56. Freestone JF, Beadle R, Shoemaker K, et al. Improved insulin sensitivity in hyperinsulinaemic ponies through physical conditioning and controlled feed intake. Equine Vet J 1992;24(3):187–90.

57. Powell DM, Reedy SE, Sessions DR, et al. Effect of short-term exercise training on insulin sensitivity in obese and lean mares. Equine Vet J Suppl 2002;(34):81–4.

58. Blikslager AT, Yin C, Cochran AM, et al. Cyclooxygenase expression in the early stages of equine laminitis: a cytologic study. J Vet Intern Med 2006;20(5):1191–6.

59. Stokes SM, Bertin FR, Stefanovski D, et al. The effect of continuous digital hypothermia on lamellar energy metabolism and perfusion during laminitis development in two experimental models. Equine Vet J 2020;52(4):585–92.

60. Fugler LA, Eades SC, Moore RM, et al. Plasma matrix metalloproteinase activity in horses after intravenous infusion of lipopolysaccharide and treatment with matrix metalloproteinase inhibitors. Am J Vet Res 2013;74(3):473–80.

61. Ingle-Fehr JE, Baxter GM. The effect of oral isoxsuprine and pentoxifylline on digital and laminar blood flow in healthy horses. Vet Surg 1999;28(3):154–60.

62. de Laat MA, Reiche DB, Sillence MN, et al. Incidence and risk factors for recurrence of endocrinopathic laminitis in horses. J Vet Intern Med 2019;33:1473–82.

63. Luthersson N, Mannfalk M, Parkin TDH, et al. Laminitis: risk factors and outcome in a group of Danish horses. J Equine Vet Sci 2017;53:68–73.

64. McGowan CM, Frost R, Pfeiffer DU, et al. Serum insulin concentrations in horses with equine Cushing's syndrome: response to a cortisol inhibitor and prognostic value. Equine Vet J 2004;36(3):295–8.

Laminitis Updates
Sepsis/Systemic Inflammatory Response Syndrome–Associated Laminitis

Britta Sigrid Leise, DVM, PhD*, Lee Ann Fugler, DVM, PhD

KEYWORDS

- Horse • Systemic inflammatory response syndrome • Inflammatory mediators
- Cytokines • Therapies

KEY POINTS

- Experimental models of sepsis/systemic inflammatory response syndrome (SIRS)-associated laminitis have helped to elucidate the pathophysiological mechanisms of inflammation and their signaling cascades. This information will further advance the development of preventative therapies for this devastating disease.

- Prolonged and sustained systemic inflammatory response may increase the risk and severity of laminitis in horses with SIRS; therefore, rapid identification and initiation of preventative measure are recommended.

- Although there are several preventative therapies that can be used in the horse with SIRS, digital hypothermia (also known as cryotherapy) is the one anti-inflammatory therapy with extensive evidence to support its use clinically. Anti-inflammatory effects of cryotherapy are the greatest when applied before the development of lameness.

INTRODUCTION

Laminitis is a severely debilitating, life-threatening disorder affecting the dermal and epidermal tissues of the equine digit (**Table 1**). The development of laminitis occurs as a sequela to many clinical conditions in the horse, including various gastrointestinal disorders, pneumonia, metritis, and grain overload. Many of these disorders elicit a severe inflammatory response known as systemic inflammatory response syndrome (SIRS). SIRS may result from an infectious process that enters the circulation (sepsis) or can result from trigger factors produced/released by injured or damaged tissues. Uncontrolled SIRS can lead to organ failure, which is most often manifested in the horse as laminitis. Acute laminitis is also associated with the endocrine conditions equine metabolic syndrome (EMS) and pituitary pars intermedia

Department of Veterinary Clinical Sciences, Louisiana State University, School of Veterinary Medicine, Baton Rouge, LA 70803, USA
* Corresponding author.
E-mail address: bleise@lsu.edu

Vet Clin Equine 37 (2021) 639–656
https://doi.org/10.1016/j.cveq.2021.08.003
0749-0739/21/Published by Elsevier Inc.

vetequine.theclinics.com

Table 1
Equine systemic inflammatory response syndrome criteria[17]

	SIRS Criteria
Heart rate	>52 bpm
Respiratory rate	>20 bpm
Rectal temperature	>101.3°F or <98.6°F
White blood cell count	>12.5 × 10⁹ cells/L or <5 × 10⁹ cells/L

dysfunction (see Nora S. Grenager's article, "Endocrinopathic laminitis," in this issue.) and may occur secondary to mechanical overload owing to severe support limb (contralateral) lameness (see Andrew van Eps and colleagues' article, "Supporting Limb Laminitis," in this issue.).[1,2] Because many diverse conditions are associated with the development of laminitis, the pathogenesis is likely complex. Although researchers have attempted to discover 1 unifying theory regarding the pathogenesis of this devastating disease in the horse, it has become increasingly clear that the numerous proposed mechanisms are most likely interconnected.[3,4] An improved understanding of the pathophysiologic mechanisms involved in the development of laminitis can enhance the ability of clinicians to prevent its onset; however, it remains a challenge to successfully treat laminitic horses once clinical signs appear. Therefore, early and aggressive therapies are recommended in horses at risk for the development of sepsis/SIRS-related laminitis.

PATHOPHYSIOLOGY OF SYSTEMIC INFLAMMATORY RESPONSE SYNDROME

SIRS refers to the uncontrolled inflammatory processes that occur following the host's response to pathogens, pathogen-associated molecular patterns (PAMPs), or damage associated molecular patterns (DAMPs).[5] Although SIRS can occur in both infectious and noninfectious diseases, it is often a sequela to sepsis owing to the liberation of bacteria and PAMPs released into the circulation during the septic state. Dysregulation of the inflammatory response, dysregulated coagulation, increased cellular death, and energy loss through mitochondrial dysfunction all play roles in SIRS. The presence of a pathogen, PAMP, or DAMP triggers the innate immune system by recruiting phagocytes to the effector site (**Fig. 1**). Production of proinflammatory cytokines by phagocytes and other effector cells, such as endothelial and epithelial cells, results in the upregulation of adhesion molecules, chemokines, and additional inflammatory cytokines (see **Fig. 1**). Leukocyte migration to the lamellae and other organs occurs during SIRS in the horse. Although essential for eradication of pathogens and injured cells, the release of reactive oxygen species (ROS) and proteases by leukocytes and other cells can injure surrounding tissue and subsequently precipitate a worsening of the inflammatory response.

MULTIORGAN DYSFUNCTION SYNDROME

The profound systemic inflammatory effects of SIRS can lead to remote organ dysfunction and the development of multiorgan dysfunction syndrome (MODS; see **Fig. 1**). Typical organs involved in MODS include, but are not limited to, the heart, lungs, kidney, and liver.[6] In the horse, the primary remote "organ" to fail is the lamellae of the hoof, resulting in the development of laminitis[7]; therefore, specific therapies targeting the developmental stage of laminitis should be used and are discussed later in

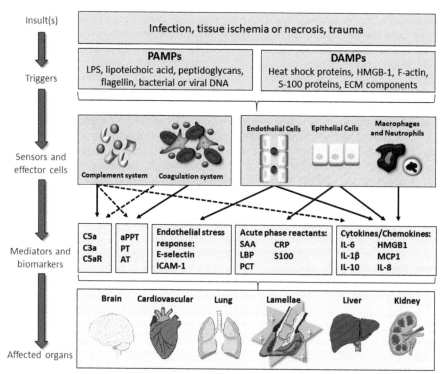

Fig. 1. SIRS pathway from insult to activation of immune and effector cells to overall effects on multiple organs. Experimental models have shown that the inflammatory response in the lamellae is greater than other organs, such as the liver, lung, and kidney, and therefore, is the most likely to fail in patients with SIRS. aPPT, activated partial thromboplastin clotting time; AT, antithrombin 3; CRP, C-reactive protein; ECM, extracellular matrix; LBP, lipopolysaccharide binding protein; PT, prothrombin. (*Adapted from* Reinhart et al.; Clin Microbiol Rev (2012) 25:610.)

this article. Advancement of SIRS to MODS indicates severe illness, significantly complicating treatment and decreasing the patient's prognosis for survival.[8,9]

EXPERIMENTAL MODELS OF SYSTEMIC INFLAMMATORY RESPONSE SYNDROME–ASSOCIATED LAMINITIS

There are 3 well-known experimental models used to study SIRS-associated laminitis. One of the first experimental laminitis models developed was the carbohydrate overload (CHO) model,[10] which was established to mimic grain overload in the horse.[10,11] In this model, horses receive a 17.6 g/kg mixture of corn starch (85%) and wood flour (15%) via nasogastric intubation. Microbial alterations in the cecum result in decreased pH, an increased number of gram-positive bacteria, death of gram-negative bacteria followed by liberation of endotoxin, and substantial mucosal disruption with an increase in permeability.[12–14] This results in a systemic inflammatory process, exhibited clinically by fever, diarrhea, colic, and dehydration 12 to 20 hours post-CHO administration. Onset of clinical Obel grade 1 laminitis occurs 24 to 48 hours post-CHO administration, and Obel grade 3 laminitis occurs between 40 and 72 hours post-CHO administration.[10,11,15] A more recent carbohydrate model has been developed to mimic laminitis resulting from ingestion of fructans in lush pasture. This model uses the administration of the nonstructural carbohydrate, oligofructose (OF), which is extracted from the roots of chicory and is administered at 5 to 10 g/kg of body weight via nasogastric intubation.[16,17] Administration of OF results in self-limiting diarrhea with electrolytes and fluid losses similar to that seen in horses with colitis.[17] Changes in cecal flora and production of endotoxin also occur in this model.[17,18] Clinical signs of Obel grade 1 laminitis occur approximately 20 to 30 hours post-OF administration. The last experimental model of SIRS-associated laminitis is the black walnut extract (BWE) model, which was developed from the observation that horses bedded on black walnut shavings would commonly develop laminitis.[19] Horses are administered BWE at 2 g/kg of body weight via nasogastric intubation that is obtained by soaking shavings from the heartwood of a black walnut tree. A classic drop in circulating white blood cells (WBC; leukopenia) occurs 3 to 4 hours post-BWE administration followed by relatively rapid onset of lameness at 10 to 12 hours post-BWE administration.[20] Although this model has a rapid onset of lameness with mild side effects, gross evidence of lamellar destruction/failure rarely occurs when compared with the CHO and OF models.[21] Differences between the carbohydrate models and BWE model have similarities to models of sepsis studied in mice. The BWE model closely mimics intraperitoneal administration of endotoxin, resulting in a rapid, intense peak of inflammation, whereas the CHO model more closely mimics the polymicrobial cecal ligation and puncture model, resulting in a prolonged and sustained inflammatory response (**Fig. 2**). Duration and severity of the inflammatory response is the main difference between these models,[20,22] suggesting that a prolonged systemic inflammatory response is more likely to result in severe disease.

Several studies have been conducted using these experimental models to determine the pathophysiology of sepsis/SIRS-associated laminitis. Administration of CHO, OF, or BWE via nasogastric intubation results in alterations within the gastrointestinal tract, including changes in microbial flora, injury to mucosa, and increased permeability of PAMPs and DAMPs followed by their release into the circulation.

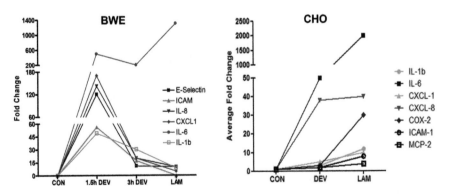

Fig. 2. Cytokine and chemokine gene expression in the lamellae of horses with BWE-induced laminitis and CHO-induced laminitis. The peak of expression is early in the developmental period within the lamellar tissue of horses receiving BWE and is later at the onset of lameness in horses receiving CHO. The intense rapid peak with BWE is like a rapid infusion of endotoxin, whereas the CHO administration results in a slower onset but longer effect. This prolonged inflammatory effect results in more severe lamellar injury in this model and more closely mimics that of clinical cases with sepsis or SIRS. CON, control; DEV, developmental time point; ICAM, intercellular adhesion molecule-1; LAM, onset of lameness.

Circulation of these PAMPs and DAMPs extends to systemic organs, such as the liver, lung, and kidney, and results in systemic inflammation. Interestingly, horses that did not develop a systemic inflammatory response after administration of CHO or OF also did not develop laminitis.[22,23] This suggests limiting or preventing SIRS prevents the development of laminitis. Although there are some differences in the overall inflammatory response between experimental models, systemic inflammation is followed by local chemokine production,[24,25] leukocyte migration,[26,27] and proinflammatory mediator production within the digital lamellae.[22,28] Furthermore, expression of proinflammatory mediators, such as interleukin-1β (IL-1β), stimulates the production and activation of extracellular matrix proteases (eg, matrix metalloproteinase [MMPs]) that result in breakdown of the basement membrane and the lamellar keratinocyte attachments. The addition of mechanical stress through weight bearing further stretches and tears the injured lamellar tissue, thereby ultimately resulting in lamellar failure.

SIGNALING PATHWAYS INVOLVED IN SEPSIS/SYSTEMIC INFLAMMATORY RESPONSE SYNDROME–ASSOCIATED LAMINITIS

Multiple signaling pathways are involved in the development of sepsis/SIRS-associated laminitis. Interaction of these pathways results in redundancies of complex mechanisms and consequently causes dysregulation of the inflammatory response in various disease states.

The initiation of SIRS begins with the recognition of infective agents and/or injured cells through toll-like receptor (TLR) binding of PAMPs and DAMPs, respectively. Cells of the innate immune system as well as epithelial cells in various organs possess TLRs, which bind conserved molecular structures of pathogens and damage-associated proteins.[29] Of the 10 TLRs known, the first and best described is TLR-4, which binds lipopolysaccharide (LPS) from gram-negative bacteria.[30] Initial exposure to LPS results in binding of the lipid A portion of the LPS molecule to a LPS binding protein (**Fig. 3**).[31] This, along with CD14, facilitates binding to the TLR-4 receptor.

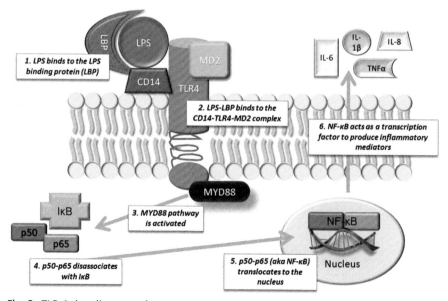

Fig. 3. TLR-4 signaling cascade.

Downstream signaling cascades are activated, and nuclear factor-κB (NF-κB) is subsequently translocated to the nucleus, where it stimulates transcription of more than 40 different proinflammatory genes (see **Fig. 3**). Increased expression of TLR-2 and TLR-4 has been found in the lamellar epithelial basal cells of horses with CHO-induced laminitis.[28]

The signal transducing activators of transcription factors (STATs) are latent intracytoplasmic proteins that when activated are translocated to the nucleus to produce various inflammatory genes.[32] Phosphorylation or activation of STATs can occur by several different pathways. The best-described pathway is the Janus kinase (JAK)-STAT pathway, which is activated through cytokine (eg, IL-6) binding of a cell surface receptor (**Fig. 4**).[33] Cytokine binding results in apposition of 2 JAK proteins, which are subsequently phosphorylated. STAT proteins are then activated and form dimers, which are translocated to the nucleus, to serve as transcription factors for the production of proinflammatory mediators.[34,35] Although activation of both STAT1 and STAT3 has been reported in models of human sepsis/SIRS,[36–38] only STAT3 activation was seen in the laminae from the CHO and BWE models of laminitis.[39] The authors suspect that the predominate stimulator of STAT3 activation was due to IL-6, as a profound increase in messenger RNA expression is known to affect the lamellae in experimental models.

An alternative pathway of gp130/IL-6 receptor binding is through PI3K-mTOR signaling. Binding of IL-6 to the IL-6/gp130 receptor results in a series of downstream phosphorylation events (**Fig. 5**) of Akt, mTOR, and RPS6.[40] Phosphorylation of ribosome protein, RPS6, at the serine moieties results in the translation of proteins

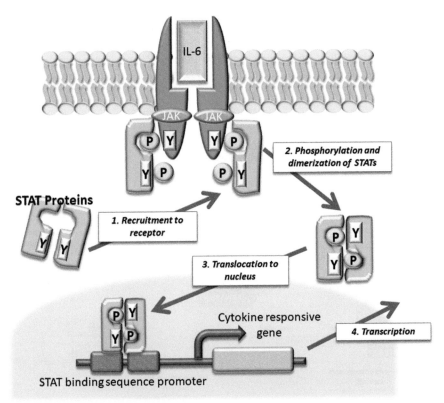

Fig. 4. IL-6/gp130 signaling through STAT3 activation.

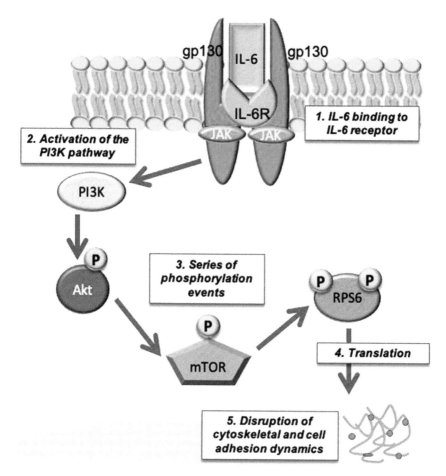

Fig. 5. IL-6/gp130 signaling through PI3K-mTOR activation.

regulating cytoskeletal structure and cell adhesion dynamics. Lamellar concentrations of signaling proteins downstream of IL-6/gp130, through the PI3K pathway, were increased post-OF administration.[40] Application of digital hypothermia resulted in downregulation of mTOR-RPS6 signaling, demonstrating a potential mechanism for the protective effects cryotherapy exerts on the digital lamellae.[40] Interestingly, the PI3K pathway has also been reported to be activated secondary to IGF-1 receptor binding of insulin. This finding supports a common mechanism of cytoskeletal dysregulation and cell adhesion disruption. Inhibitors of this pathway may provide additional therapies for the prevention of sepsis/SIRS-associated laminitis in the future.

EVALUATION OF THE SEPSIS/SYSTEMIC INFLAMMATORY RESPONSE SYNDROME PATIENT

The presence of sepsis/SIRS in equine patients has been associated with the development of laminitis[7]; therefore, rapid identification of sepsis/SIRS allows for prompt initiation of therapeutic measures to limit inflammation and prevent lamellar injury.

The presence of a fever along with an increase in WBC count (with or without the presence of band neutrophils) and hyperfibrinogenemia is often associated with infection but may also be present with noninfectious inflammatory diseases. A definitive diagnosis of sepsis is made when a microorganism (such as bacteria or virus) has been isolated. The clinical definition for SIRS in the horse has been extrapolated from examination parameters described in humans (**Table 1**).[5] An equine patient is considered to have SIRS if at least 2 of the following 4 parameters are present: (1) heart rate greater than 52 bpm, (2) respiratory rate greater than 20 bpm, (3) rectal temperature less than 98.6°F or greater than 101.3°F, and (4) WBC count less than 5×10^9 cells/L or greater than 12.5×10^9 cells/L.[9] In 1 study, adult horses with an SIRS score of 3 or 4 out of 4 had an increased risk of death compared with those with lower scores.[9]

In addition to the parameters used to identify the presence of SIRS in the horse, other clinical findings that have been associated with endotoxemia include hemoconcentration (indicated by increased packed-cell volume (PCV)/total protein (TP)), hyperemic or toxic mucous membranes with prolonged capillary refill time, and hyperlactemia.[9,41] The presence and severity of these findings have been reported to be associated with outcome. In 1 retrospective study, horses with signs of endotoxemia were 5 times more likely to develop laminitis when hospitalized than horses without clinical signs.[41]

Biomarkers of sepsis and SIRS have been studied intensely in humans with more than 170 different compounds evaluated for their diagnostic and prognostic abilities.[42] Nevertheless, despite numerous studies, the ideal biomarker has yet to be identified. Experimentally induced SIRS-associated laminitis has identified the upregulation of numerous proinflammatory cytokines within the lamellar tissue, including IL-6, IL-1β, and cyclooxygenase-2 (COX-2).[22] Circulating inflammatory mediators and biomarkers have been more challenging to identify because of difficulties in obtaining equine-specific reagents. However, serum amyloid A (SAA), procalcitonin (PCT), and calprotectin have been identified as potential markers for SIRS in the horse.[43,44]

SAA is an acute phase protein released into the circulation, mainly by the liver, in response to inflammatory and infectious stimuli. Circulating levels of SAA are usually low or unmeasurable, but can increase rapidly in less than 4 hours when induced by IL-1β and reach maximal levels in 24 to 48 hours.[45] SAA was found to be significantly increased in horses with SIRS secondary to gastrointestinal disease.[43]

PCT can be secreted by numerous cell types in response to inflammation.[44] Because of its rapid increase in plasma concentrations and relatively short half-life of 22 to 26 hours, it has been studied extensively as a biomarker for sepsis and other inflammatory conditions in human medicine, but has only recently begun to be investigated in veterinary medicine.[44] Although there are limited data regarding equine PCT, significant increases in plasma concentrations have been reported in horses with SIRS when compared with controls.[46] Plasma PCT concentrations were also increased in horses administered LPS as an experimental model of endotoxemia/sepsis.[47]

Calprotectin is an inflammatory protein produced mainly by neutrophils and is released into the circulation following cell disruption and death.[48] It has been used in human medicine as a biomarker for acute and chronic inflammatory diseases; however, equine calprotectin has only been studied to a small extent and is mostly limited to immunohistochemical evaluation within various tissues. Experimental models of SIRS-associated laminitis have all demonstrated increased calprotectin staining within the digital lamellae as well as in the colon of horses administered BWE.[27,49]

PREVENTIONS AND THERAPEUTICS
Treatment of the Primary Disease

As SIRS-related laminitis is a sequela to systemic inflammatory disease, a cornerstone of therapy is to halt the primary disease or condition affecting the patient and provide supportive care. Surgical correction and removal of ischemic bowel, debridement of necrotic tissue, and antibiotic therapy for known bacterial infections are examples of treatments necessary to remove the inciting cause of the systemic inflammatory response. Fluid resuscitation and maintenance of normal cardiovascular function are particularly important in horses with signs of shock; however, once the cardiovascular status is stable, judicious fluid therapy rates should be used to minimize effects of Starling forces by which excessive intravenous (IV) fluids could result in lamellar edema.

Digital Cryotherapy

Digital hypothermia, also known as cryotherapy, has been used to ameliorate experimentally induced laminitis when applied during the developmental stage and is discussed in more detail in Daniela Luethy's article, "Cryotherapy techniques – Best protocols to support the foot in health and disease," in this issue..[50–52] Suggested protocol for cryotherapy of the equine digit requires maintenance of hoof temperatures $\leq 5°C$ via submergence in an ice-water boot until the resolution of the primary disease. Continuous cryotherapy has been found experimentally to significantly reduce the expression of MMP-2[51] and numerous proinflammatory mediators within the lamellae when initiated before the onset of lameness.[53] Cryotherapy also decreased expression of chemotactic mediators, which subsequently prevented leukocyte migration into the lamellae after OF administration.[53] However, when delayed until the onset of lameness, the anti-inflammatory effects of cryotherapy were not noted despite its ability to minimize histologic changes within the lamellae.[54] In addition to experimental evidence, cryotherapy, when used prophylactically, has also been reported to decrease the incidence of laminitis in clinical cases of SIRS.[55]

Nonsteroidal Anti-Inflammatories

It is well documented that the lamellae of the equine digit demonstrates a strong proinflammatory response to systemic disease. In particular, an increase in COX-2 expression has been reported to occur with experimentally induced SIRS-associated laminitis.[22,56] Nonsteroidal anti-inflammatory drugs (NSAIDs) by far are one of the most common therapies used in the treatment and prevention of laminitis. In an epidemiologic study of laminitis,[57] it was reported that 68% of cases were treated with phenylbutazone and 19% of cases were treated with flunixin meglumine. Despite their common use, only minimal lamellar protection was achieved with phenylbutazone or flunixin meglumine when used as a sole treatment in a model of CHO-induced laminitis.[58] Typical doses for phenylbutazone range between 2.2 mg/kg and 4.4 mg/kg of body weight administered orally or IV every 12 to 24 hours. Doses for flunixin meglumine range from 0.25 mg/kg of body weight IV every 8 hours to 1.1 mg/kg of body weight IV every 12 hours. Both phenylbutazone and flunixin meglumine are COX-1 and COX-2 inhibitors and therefore have the potential to induce side effects associated with COX-1 inhibition, including gastrointestinal ulceration and renal papillary necrosis. Firocoxib, an equine COX-2-specific NSAID, has potential benefits over the traditional NSAIDs, by decreasing the risk of gastrointestinal side effects while still blocking COX-2 activity within the lamellar tissue. However, negative cardiovascular effects have been associated with the use of COX-2-specific inhibitors in humans. Because of this, there has been some question regarding the use of firocoxib early in the developmental stages of laminitis.[59] It is unknown what affects firocoxib may have on the balance of thromboxane-A2 and prostacyclin at the level of the lamellar vessels. A shift in this balance could possibly result in procoagulative state, thereby increasing the risk of thrombi formation, which could adversely affect patients with laminitis. Despite this concern, many clinicians use firocoxib in both acute and chronic cases of laminitis for both its anti-inflammatory and its pain-relieving effects. The reported recommended dosage for firocoxib is 0.1 mg/kg orally every 24 hours.

Polymyxin B

Polymyxin B, a cationic polypeptide antibiotic, binds the lipid-A portion of LPS and neutralizes the actions of endotoxin in vitro.[60] It also neutralizes the gram-positive toxins lipoteichoic acid (LTA) and peptidoglycan, demonstrated by decreased tumor necrosis factor-α (TNF-α) activity in equine whole blood stimulated by these mediators.[61] Nephrotoxicity is possible when polymyxin B is used at the antimicrobial dose; however, polymyxin B exerts antiendotoxic effects at serum concentrations substantially lower than those required for antimicrobial effectiveness. Clinically, polymyxin B is administered to horses at a dosage of 6000 U/kg[60] IV every 8 to 12 hours diluted in 1 L of saline. Typically, this therapy is continued for up to 5 treatments or until the signs of endotoxemia subside. Although polymyxin B administered at 6000 U/kg IV every 8 hours did not accumulate in the vasculature and had no effect on urine GGT-to-creatinine ratio,[60] caution should be used in horses that are obviously dehydrated, hypovolemic, or azotemic until these abnormalities are corrected. Polymyxin B has been reported to have its greatest effect when given before endotoxin release[62]; therefore, it should ideally be administered early in the course of treatment, particularly in cases whereby reperfusion and/or microbial death may occur secondarily to management of the primary disease. However, even when administered after the onset of endotoxemia, polymyxin B significantly reduced fever, tachycardia, and serum TNF-α concentrations.[62]

Pentoxifylline

Pentoxifylline (PTX) is a phosphodiesterase inhibitor used by clinicians in the treatment of laminitis for its rheologic and anti-inflammatory effects. PTX improves capillary blood flow by reducing blood viscosity and increasing erythrocyte deformability. Its anti-inflammatory effects most likely result from decreased inflammatory mediator transcription because of its ability to inhibit phosphodiesterase and increase intracellular cyclic adenosine monophosphate.[63] These effects include decreased cytokine expression and release, neutrophil inhibition, and decreased ROS synthesis and activity. The ability of PTX to inhibit TNF-α and other inflammatory cytokines suggests that it may be an effective treatment for endotoxemia/SIRS. In an in vitro model of endotoxemia, PTX decreased TNF-α and IL-6 concentrations in whole blood exposed to LPS.[64] This occurred in a dose-dependent manner regardless of PTX treatment time in regard to the addition of LPS; however, tissue factor activity was inhibited only with pretreatment of PTX.[64] PTX also had an inhibitory effect on LPS-induced equine neutrophil activation ex vivo, evident by decreased CD11/CD18 expression.[65] In vivo PTX administration for the treatment of experimental endotoxemia yields varying results. When given post-LPS administration, PTX had little effect on the inflammatory variables measured, although it did decrease rectal temperature, respiratory rate, and whole blood recalcification time.[66] In another study, PTX administered before the induction of endotoxemia decreased plasminogen activator inhibitor-1 concentrations and increased prostacyclin concentrations; however, PTX had no effect on TNF-α or IL-6 concentrations.[67] MMP activity, which is thought to play an important role in basement membrane breakdown between the lamellar dermal-epidermal interface, increases during inflammation, resulting in tissue destruction and further activation of proinflammatory mediators. Endotoxin-induced MMP-2 and -9 activity in horses was significantly decreased by the administration of PTX,[68] and in a preliminary report, PTX was also found to decrease the severity of CHO-induced laminitis when compared with controls[69]; therefore, PTX has been recommended as a therapeutic for the prevention of laminitis in horses with SIRS. Dosages for PTX vary; however, 1 study found PTX reached plasma concentrations equivalent to therapeutic doses in people when administered at 10 mg/kg orally every 12 hours.[70] Clinically, a dosage range of 8.5 to 10 mg/kg orally every 8 to 12 hours is commonly used. PTX may also be administered slowly IV at a dose of 8.5 mg/kg every 8 to 12 hours.

Dimethyl Sulfoxide

Dimethyl sulfoxide (DMSO) is administered to horses for its putative anti-inflammatory effects related to its ability to scavenge oxygen free radicals. Administration of high-dose DMSO (1 g/kg) attenuated endotoxin-induced fever experimentally; however, no other significant changes were reported in heart rate, respiratory rate, WBC count, blood glucose concentration, or blood lactate concentration after DMSO administration at either the high (1 g/kg IV) or the low (20 mg/kg IV) dose.[71] One retrospective study found that DMSO was used in 27% of laminitic cases,[57] despite that no controlled studies have been reported to support definitive benefits of this therapy. The lack of benefit may be due to the fact that little evidence of oxidant stress has been found during the developmental phases of laminitis.[72]

Clopidogrel, Aspirin, and Heparin

Systemic inflammation can lead to activation of coagulation and downregulation of anticoagulant pathways and subsequent thrombin production.[73] In addition, activation of coagulation can influence endothelial and inflammatory cell function, thereby further affecting inflammatory activity. Horses with SIRS have been reported to have significantly lower platelet counts compared with horses without SIRS; however, in that study there was no difference in platelet aggregation.[74] Increased platelet aggregation and plasma LPS concentrations have been reported in horses 8 to 12 hours post-OF administration.[75] Treatment with a platelet fibrinogen receptor antagonist in ponies administered CHO ameliorated the production of platelet-neutrophil aggregates and prevented the development of laminitis.[76] Based on this study, therapeutics that inhibit activation of coagulation may be beneficial in the prevention of sepsis/SIRS-related laminitis.

Administration of clopidogrel, an antagonist of the platelet $P2Y_{12}$ adenosine diphosphate receptor, has been reported to inhibit platelet aggregation in normal horses but did not affect serotonin release.[77] This inhibition of platelet function was prolonged, continuing 6 days postadministration, suggesting that the effects of clopidogrel are irreversible.[77] Clopidogrel is administered to horses at a loading dose of 6 to 6.5 mg/kg of body weight followed by 2.0 mg/kg PO every 24 hours. Although clopidogrel appears to have benefits in inhibiting platelet aggregation in normal horses, its effects on horses with SIRS and its ability to prevent the development of laminitis have yet to be determined. Other medications that have been purportedly used for their antithrombotic effects include aspirin (10–20 mg/kg orally every 48 hours) and heparin (40–80 IU/kg IV or subcutaneously every 8 hours). Although aspirin administration decreases thromboxane production in normal horses, platelet aggregation was not inhibited.[77] Low-molecular-weight heparin downregulates the prothrombotic state and has been reported to decrease the prevalence of laminitis in postoperative colics.[78]

Lidocaine and Ketamine

Lidocaine and ketamine may be used in horses with laminitis for their analgesic effects but also have potential anti-inflammatory benefits in some species. Conflicting results regarding the anti-inflammatory effects of lidocaine in horses exist. Experimentally, lidocaine given as a constant rate infusion of 0.05 mg/kg/min decreased clinical signs of endotoxemia and TNF-α concentrations in the peritoneal fluid of horses after intraperitoneal administration of LPS. However, neutrophil migration and adhesion were not inhibited by therapeutic concentrations of lidocaine in vitro.[79] In addition, systemic administration of lidocaine to horses with BWE-induced laminitis did not affect leukocyte migration into the lamellar tissue or inflammatory mediator expression within the lamellae.[80] Although lidocaine's anti-inflammatory effects are questionable, its use for pain management in clinical cases of laminitis may have some benefits.

Ketamine, a dissociative anesthetic and NMDA receptor antagonist, has immunomodulating effects on endotoxin-induced shock in rats.[81] Inhibition of NF-κB signaling and subsequent decreased pro-inflammatory cytokine expression have been reported in equine cell lines after LPS exposure.[82] However, horses receiving subanesthetic doses of ketamine (loading dose of 2.4 mg/kg/h followed by CRI of 1.5 mg/kg/h for a total infusion period of 6 hours) did not demonstrate improved clinical signs or inflammatory parameters after LPS infusion.[83] In addition, transient excitation was noted during administration of the loading dose; therefore, further study is needed to determine if ketamine has significant in vivo anti-inflammatory effects before being used for this purpose clinically.

Leukapheresis

Leukapheresis, the process of removing leukocytes from the systemic circulation, has been evaluated in horses with experimentally induced SIRS.[84] Four hours of apheresis resulted in 31% reduction in neutrophils and 59% reduction in monocytes from the circulation compared with basal values.[84] Clinically, horses receiving leukapheresis before SIRS induction had significantly improved outcomes. Horses receiving leukapheresis did not develop signs of SIRS (defined by tachycardia and hyperthermia) or MODS (defined by increased blood concentrations of glucose, creatinine, and liver enzymes).[85] Although they are currently only used experimentally, findings from this study suggest that mechanisms to reduce leukocyte activity (such as IL-8 inhibitors) may improve outcomes in horses with SIRS.

Mechanical Support

Mechanical stabilization of the forces placed on the digit is essential to limit injury to the lamellar tissue during sepsis or SIRS. Treatment of local and systemic inflammation may not be enough to prevent some lamellar injury from occurring, and weight-bearing forces should be minimized to prevent further damage. It is important to neutralize these forces appropriately, and methods used should be tailored to the individual patient. More information on mechanical support can be found Raul Bras and Scott Morrison's article, "Mechanical Principles of the Equine Foot," in this issue, and Andrew van Eps and colleagues' article, "Supporting Limb Laminitis," in this issue.

Novel Therapies

Although the inflammatory response accompanying the development of sepsis/SIRS-associated laminitis is well documented and recent studies have elucidated several downstream signaling markers (eg, NF-κB, STAT3, and mTOR), there remains potential therapies that have yet to be evaluated for their ability to prevent the development and treat laminitis in the horse. For example, the use of STAT3 inhibitors has been found to improve survivability in a cecal ligation puncture model of sepsis.[86] In contrast, other reports suggest that STAT3 activation is necessary for the liver to mount an appropriate immune response in the face of sepsis.[87,88] These mixed reports suggest that more research is needed before determining if STAT3 inhibitors would result in beneficial effects when treating sepsis/SIRS-associated laminitis. Another exciting, potential therapeutic drug is the mTOR inhibitor, rapamycin. Rapamycin inhibition of serine phosphorylation was found to protect epithelial structural integrity through the preservation of desmosomal adhesion. As downstream activation of mTOR has been reported in both the sepsis/SIRS model and endocrine model of laminitis, inhibitors of this signaling pathway may have benefit in laminitis resulting from varying causes.[40] In addition to downstream signaling inhibitors, IL-6 receptor antagonist may also provide potential therapeutic benefits. Lamellar expression of IL-6 during sepsis/SIRS-associated laminitis is overwhelming[22] and is followed by both STAT3 and PI3K-mTOR signaling.[40] Inhibition of IL-6 could theoretically prevent downstream signaling and prevent cytoskeletal dysregulation and subsequently lamellar failure. Monoclonal antibodies developed to block IL-6 have been used in people with sepsis/SIRS with varying results. However, IL-6 signaling is complex having a membrane-bound (eg,"classical") as well as a soluble (eg, "trans") receptor. Unfortunately, further studies are needed to determine how these 2 varying components are affected by receptor antagonists in the horse before the development of new therapies.

CLINICS CARE POINTS

- Diagnosis of SIRS in the horse can be made based off of clinical findings including: temperature, heart rate, respiratory rate, and total white blood cell count.
- Laminitis is a common sequela to SIRS in the horse.
- Laminitis preventions, such as digital cryotherapy, anti-inflammatory medications, and anti-endotoxic therapies should be initiated early in the course of SIRS and continued throughout until clinical signs have resolved.
- Research has recently revealed a potential common signaling pathway (mTOR) that may allow the development of new therapies that can be directed towards preventing and treating laminitis in the future.

DISCLOSURE

The authors have no conflicts of interest to disclose.

REFERENCES

1. Baxter GM. Acute laminitis. Vet Clin North Am Equine Pract 1994;10(3):627–42.
2. Baxter GM, Morrison S. Complications of unilateral weight bearing. Vet Clin North Am Equine Pract 2008;24(3). 621-642, ix.
3. Eades SC. Overview of current laminitis research. Vet Clin North Am Equine Pract 2010;26(1):51–63.

4. van Eps AW, Burns TA. Are there shared mechanisms in the pathophysiology of different clinical forms of laminitis and what are the implications for prevention and treatment? Vet Clin North Am Equine Pract 2019;35(2):379–98.

5. Bone RC, Balk RA, Cerra FB, et al. Definitions for sepsis and organ failure and guidelines for the use of innovative therapies in sepsis. The ACCP/SCCM Consensus Conference Committee. American College of Chest Physicians/Society of Critical Care Medicine. Chest 1992;101(6):1644–55.

6. Sheats MK. A comparative review of equine SIRS, sepsis, and neutrophils. Front Vet Sci 2019;6:69.

7. Belknap JK, Moore JN, Crouser EC. Sepsis-from human organ failure to laminar failure. Vet Immunol Immunopathol 2009;129(3–4):155–7.

8. McConachie E, Giguere S, Barton MH. Scoring system for multiple organ dysfunction in adult horses with acute surgical gastrointestinal disease. J Vet Intern Med 2016;30(4):1276–83.

9. Roy MF, Kwong GP, Lambert J, et al. Prognostic value and development of a scoring system in horses with systemic inflammatory response syndrome. J Vet Intern Med 2017;31(2):582–92.

10. Garner HE, Coffman JR, Hahn AW, et al. Equine laminitis of alimentary origin: an experimental model. Am J Vet Res 1975;36(4 Pt.1):441–4.

11. Allen D Jr, Clark ES, Moore JN, et al. Evaluation of equine digital Starling forces and hemodynamics during early laminitis. Am J Vet Res 1990;51(12):1930–4.

12. Garner HE, Moore JN, Johnson JH, et al. Changes in the caecal flora associated with the onset of laminitis. Equine Vet J 1978;10(4):249–52.

13. Krueger AS, Kinden DA, Garner HE, et al. Ultrastructural study of the equine cecum during onset of laminitis. Am J Vet Res 1986;47(8):1804–12.

14. Moore JN, Garner HE, Berg JN, et al. Intracecal endotoxin and lactate during the onset of equine laminitis: a preliminary report. Am J Vet Res 1979;40(5):722–3.

15. Moore JN, Allen D Jr, Clark ES. Pathophysiology of acute laminitis. Vet Clin North Am Equine Pract 1989;5(1):67–72.

16. Kalck KA, Frank N, Elliott SB, et al. Effects of low-dose oligofructose treatment administered via nasogastric intubation on induction of laminitis and associated alterations in glucose and insulin dynamics in horses. Am J Vet Res 2009; 70(5):624–32.

17. van Eps AW, Pollitt CC. Equine laminitis induced with oligofructose. Equine Vet J 2006;38(3):203–8.

18. Milinovich GJ, Trott DJ, Burrell PC, et al. Changes in equine hindgut bacterial populations during oligofructose-induced laminitis. Environ Microbiol 2006;8(5): 885–98.

19. Uhlinger C. Black walnut toxicosis in ten horses. J Am Vet Med Assoc 1989; 195(3):343–4.

20. Belknap JK, Giguere S, Pettigrew A, et al. Lamellar pro-inflammatory cytokine expression patterns in laminitis at the developmental stage and at the onset of lameness: innate vs. adaptive immune response. Equine Vet J 2007;39(1):42–7.

21. Pollitt CC. Basement membrane pathology: a feature of acute equine laminitis. Equine Vet J 1996;28(1):38–46.

22. Leise BS, Faleiros RR, Watts M, et al. Laminar inflammatory gene expression in the carbohydrate overload model of equine laminitis. Equine Vet J 2011;43(1): 54–61.

23. Tadros EM, Frank N, Newkirk KM, et al. Effects of a "two-hit" model of organ damage on the systemic inflammatory response and development of laminitis in horses. Vet Immunol Immunopathol 2012;150(1–2):90–100.

24. Faleiros RR, Leise BS, Watts M, et al. Laminar chemokine mRNA concentrations in horses with carbohydrate overload-induced laminitis. Vet Immunol Immunopathol 2011;144(1–2):45–51.

25. Faleiros RR, Leise BB, Westerman T, et al. In vivo and in vitro evidence of the involvement of CXCL1, a keratinocyte-derived chemokine, in equine laminitis. J Vet Intern Med 2009;23(5):1086–96.

26. Faleiros RR, Johnson PJ, Nuovo GJ, et al. Laminar leukocyte accumulation in horses with carbohydrate overload-induced laminitis. J Vet Intern Med 2011; 25(1):107–15.

27. Faleiros RR, Nuovo GJ, Belknap JK. Calprotectin in myeloid and epithelial cells of laminae from horses with black walnut extract-induced laminitis. J Vet Intern Med 2009;23(1):174–81.

28. Leise BS, Watts MR, Roy S, et al. Use of laser capture microdissection for the assessment of equine lamellar basal epithelial cell signalling in the early stages of laminitis. Equine Vet J 2015;47(4):478–88.

29. Janssens S, Beyaert R. Role of toll-like receptors in pathogen recognition. Clin Microbiol Rev 2003;16(4):637–46.

30. Chaudhary PM, Ferguson C, Nguyen V, et al. Cloning and characterization of two toll/interleukin-1 receptor-like genes TIL3 and TIL4: evidence for a multi-gene receptor family in humans. Blood 1998;91(11):4020–7.

31. Palsson-McDermott EM, O'Neill LA. Signal transduction by the lipopolysaccharide receptor, toll-like receptor-4. Immunology 2004;113(2):153–62.

32. Levy DE, Darnell JE Jr. Stats: transcriptional control and biological impact. Nat Rev Mol Cell Biol 2002;3(9):651–62.

33. Greenlund AC, Morales MO, Viviano BL, et al. Stat recruitment by tyrosine-phosphorylated cytokine receptors: an ordered reversible affinity-driven process. Immunity 1995;2(6):677–87.

34. Lim CP, Cao X. Structure, function, and regulation of STAT proteins. Mol Biosyst 2006;2(11):536–50.

35. Reich NC, Liu L. Tracking STAT nuclear traffic. Nat Rev Immunol 2006;6(8): 602–12.

36. Kumar A, Michael P, Brabant D, et al. Human serum from patients with septic shock activates transcription factors STAT1, IRF1, and NF-kappaB and induces apoptosis in human cardiac myocytes. J Biol Chem 2005;280(52):42619–26.

37. Matsukawa A. STAT proteins in innate immunity during sepsis: lessons from gene knockout mice. Acta Med Okayama 2007;61(5):239–45.

38. Scott MJ, Godshall CJ, Cheadle WG. Jaks, STATs, cytokines, and sepsis. Clin Diagn Lab Immunol 2002;9(6):1153–9.

39. Leise BS, Watts M, Tanhoff E, et al. Laminar regulation of STAT1 and STAT3 in black walnut extract and carbohydrate overload induced models of laminitis. J Vet Intern Med 2012;26(4):996–1004.

40. Dern K, Burns TA, Watts MR, et al. Influence of digital hypothermia on lamellar events related to IL-6/gp130 signalling in equine sepsis-related laminitis. Equine Vet J 2020;52(3):441–8.

41. Parsons CS, Orsini JA, Krafty R, et al. Risk factors for development of acute laminitis in horses during hospitalization: 73 cases (1997-2004). J Am Vet Med Assoc 2007;230(6):885–9.

42. Pierrakos C, Vincent JL. Sepsis biomarkers: a review. Crit Care 2010;14(1):R15.

43. Daniel AJ, Leise BS, Burgess BA, et al. Concentrations of serum amyloid A and plasma fibrinogen in horses undergoing emergency abdominal surgery. J Vet Emerg Crit Care (San Antonio) 2016;26(3):344–51.

44. Henriquez-Camacho C, Losa J. Biomarkers for sepsis. Biomed Res Int 2014; 2014:547818.

45. Petersen HH, Nielsen JP, Heegaard PM. Application of acute phase protein measurements in veterinary clinical chemistry. Vet Res 2004;35(2):163–87.

46. Bonelli F, Meucci V, Divers TJ, et al. Plasma procalcitonin concentration in healthy horses and horses affected by systemic inflammatory response syndrome. J Vet Intern Med 2015;29(6):1689–91.

47. Bonelli F, Meucci V, Divers TJ, et al. Kinetics of plasma procalcitonin, soluble CD14, CCL2 and IL-10 after a sublethal infusion of lipopolysaccharide in horses. Vet Immunol Immunopathol 2017;184:29–35.

48. Grosche A, Morton AJ, Graham AS, et al. Effect of large colon ischemia and reperfusion on concentrations of calprotectin and other clinicopathologic variables in jugular and colonic venous blood in horses. Am J Vet Res 2013;74(10): 1281–90.

49. Chiavaccini L, Hassel DM, Shoemaker ML, et al. Detection of calprotectin and apoptotic activity within the equine colon from horses with black walnut extract-induced laminitis. Vet Immunol Immunopathol 2011;144(3–4):366–73.

50. van Eps AW. Therapeutic hypothermia (cryotherapy) to prevent and treat acute laminitis. Vet Clin North Am Equine Pract 2010;26(1):125–33.

51. van Eps AW, Pollitt CC. Equine laminitis: cryotherapy reduces the severity of the acute lesion. Equine Vet J 2004;36(3):255–60.

52. Van Eps AW, Pollitt CC. Equine laminitis model: cryotherapy reduces the severity of lesions evaluated seven days after induction with oligofructose. Equine Vet J 2009;41(8):741–6.

53. van Eps AW, Leise BS, Watts M, et al. Digital hypothermia inhibits early lamellar inflammatory signalling in the oligofructose laminitis model. Equine Vet J 2012; 44(2):230–7.

54. Dern K, van Eps A, Wittum T, et al. Effect of continuous digital hypothermia on lamellar inflammatory signaling when applied at a clinically-relevant timepoint in the oligofructose laminitis model. J Vet Intern Med 2018;32(1):450–8.

55. Kullmann A, Holcombe SJ, Hurcombe SD, et al. Prophylactic digital cryotherapy is associated with decreased incidence of laminitis in horses diagnosed with colitis. Equine Vet J 2014;46(5):554–9.

56. Blikslager AT, Yin C, Cochran AM, et al. Cyclooxygenase expression in the early stages of equine laminitis: a cytologic study. J Vet Intern Med 2006;20(5):1191–6.

57. Slater MR, Hood DM, Carter GK. Descriptive epidemiological study of equine laminitis. Equine Vet J 1995;27(5):364–7.

58. Pase Leme F, Bonna FA, DeMarval CA, et al. Histopatologia das lâminas do casco de equinos com laminite aguda induzida e tratados com ketoprofeno, fenilbutazona e flunixin meglumine. Arq Bras Med Vet Zootec 2010;62(2):241–50.

59. Belknap JK. Pharmacology: Is there a scientific basis for anti-inflammatory therapy in laminitis. Paper presented at: 5th International Conference of Laminitis and Disease of the Foot 2008; Palm Beach, FL.

60. Morresey PR, Mackay RJ. Endotoxin-neutralizing activity of polymyxin B in blood after IV administration in horses. Am J Vet Res 2006;67(4):642–7.

61. Bauquier JR, Tudor E, Bailey SR. Anti-inflammatory effects of four potential anti-endotoxaemic drugs assessed in vitro using equine whole blood assays. J Vet Pharmacol Ther 2015;38(3):290–6.

62. Barton MH, Parviainen A, Norton N. Polymyxin B protects horses against induced endotoxaemia in vivo. Equine Vet J 2004;36(5):397–401.

63. Michetti C, Coimbra R, Hoyt DB, et al. Pentoxifylline reduces acute lung injury in chronic endotoxemia. J Surg Res 2003;115(1):92–9.

64. Barton MH, Moore JN. Pentoxifylline inhibits mediator synthesis in an equine in vitro whole blood model of endotoxemia. Circ Shock 1994;44(4):216–20.

65. Weiss DJ, Evanson OA. Evaluation of lipopolysaccharide-induced activation of equine neutrophils. Am J Vet Res 2002;63(6):811–5.

66. Barton MH, Moore JN, Norton N. Effects of pentoxifylline infusion on response of horses to in vivo challenge exposure with endotoxin. Am J Vet Res 1997;58(11):1300–7.

67. Baskett A, Barton MH, Norton N, et al. Effect of pentoxifylline, flunixin meglumine, and their combination on a model of endotoxemia in horses. Am J Vet Res 1997;58(11):1291–9.

68. Fugler LA, Eades SC, Moore RM, et al. Plasma matrix metalloproteinase activity in horses after intravenous infusion of lipopolysaccharide and treatment with matrix metalloproteinase inhibitors. Am J Vet Res 2013;74(3):473–80.

69. Fugler LA, Eades S, Koch CE, et al. Clinical and matrix metalloproteinase inhibitory effects of pentoxifyllin on carbohydrate overload laminitis: preliminary results. J Equine Vet Sci 2010;30(2):106–7.

70. Liska DA, Akucewich LH, Marsella R, et al. Pharmacokinetics of pentoxifylline and its 5-hydroxyhexyl metabolite after oral and intravenous administration of pentoxifylline to healthy adult horses. Am J Vet Res 2006;67(9):1621–7.

71. Kelmer G, Doherty TJ, Elliott S, et al. Evaluation of dimethyl sulphoxide effects on initial response to endotoxin in the horse. Equine Vet J 2008;40(4):358–63.

72. Burns TA, Westerman T, Nuovo GJ, et al. Role of oxidative tissue injury in the pathophysiology of experimentally induced equine laminitis: a comparison of 2 models. J Vet Intern Med 2011;25(3):540–8.

73. Levi M, van der Poll T. Inflammation and coagulation. Crit Care Med 2010;38(2 Suppl):S26–34.

74. Ehrmann C, Engel J, Moritz A, et al. Assessment of platelet biology in equine patients with systemic inflammatory response syndrome. J Vet Diagn Invest 2020. 1040638720983791.

75. Bailey SR, Adair HS, Reinemeyer CR, et al. Plasma concentrations of endotoxin and platelet activation in the developmental stage of oligofructose-induced laminitis. Vet Immunol Immunopathol 2009;129(3–4):167–73.

76. Weiss DJ, Evanson OA, McClenahan D, et al. Effect of a competitive inhibitor of platelet aggregation on experimentally induced laminitis in ponies. Am J Vet Res 1998;59(7):814–7.

77. Brainard BM, Epstein KL, LoBato D, et al. Effects of clopidogrel and aspirin on platelet aggregation, thromboxane production, and serotonin secretion in horses. J Vet Intern Med 2011;25(1):116–22.

78. de la Rebiere de Pouyade G, Grulke S, Detilleux J, et al. Evaluation of low-molecular-weight heparin for the prevention of equine laminitis after colic surgery. J Vet Emerg Crit Care (San Antonio) 2009;19(1):113–9.

79. Cook VL, Neuder LE, Blikslager AT, et al. The effect of lidocaine on in vitro adhesion and migration of equine neutrophils. Vet Immunol Immunopathol 2009;129(1–2):137–42.

80. Williams JM, Lin YJ, Loftus JP, et al. Effect of intravenous lidocaine administration on laminar inflammation in the black walnut extract model of laminitis. Equine Vet J 2010;42(3):261–9.

81. Taniguchi T, Takemoto Y, Kanakura H, et al. The dose-related effects of ketamine on mortality and cytokine responses to endotoxin-induced shock in rats. Anesth Analg 2003;97(6):1769–72.

82. Lankveld DP, Bull S, Van Dijk P, et al. Ketamine inhibits LPS-induced tumour necrosis factor-alpha and interleukin-6 in an equine macrophage cell line. Vet Res 2005;36(2):257–62.

83. Alcott CJ, Sponseller BA, Wong DM, et al. Clinical and immunomodulating effects of ketamine in horses with experimental endotoxemia. J Vet Intern Med 2011; 25(4):934–43.

84. Spadeto J, Olivera A, Paz C, et al. Effect of leukapheresis on the leukogram of horses subjected to a "sepsis-related" SIRS model based on oligofructose gastric administration. Equine Vet Edu 2017;29:13.

85. Spadeto J, Olivera A, Paz C, et al. Clinical effects of leukapheresis in horses subjected to a "sepsis-related" SIRS model based on oligofructose gastric adminstration. Equine Vet Edu. 2017;29:12–3.

86. Hui L, Yao Y, Wang S, et al. Inhibition of Janus kinase 2 and signal transduction and activator of transcription 3 protect against cecal ligation and puncture-induced multiple organ damage and mortality. J Trauma 2009;66(3):859–65.

87. Andrejko KM, Chen J, Deutschman CS. Intrahepatic STAT-3 activation and acute phase gene expression predict outcome after CLP sepsis in the rat. Am J Phys 1998;275(6 Pt 1):G1423–9.

88. Sakamori R, Takehara T, Ohnishi C, et al. Signal transducer and activator of transcription 3 signaling within hepatocytes attenuates systemic inflammatory response and lethality in septic mice. Hepatology 2007;46(5):1564–73.

Supporting Limb Laminitis

Andrew van Eps, BVSc, PhD, MACVSc*, Julie Engiles, BA, VMD,
Hannah Galantino-Homer, VMD, PhD

KEYWORDS

- Contralateral • Ischemia • Lamellae • Lamellar • Laminae • Laminitis
- Weight-bearing

KEY POINTS

- Supporting limb laminitis (SLL) is an important complication of conditions that cause protracted pain in one or more limbs.
- Unlike laminitis associated with sepsis or hyperinsulinemia, ischemia is a key mechanistic event in the development of SLL, and as a result, acute SLL lesions are unique.
- Rather than increased limb weight-bearing load, it appears that altered ambulatory patterns (specifically reduced limb load cycling frequency) may interfere with blood perfusion sufficiently to damage the lamellae. This damage is not confined to the supporting limb, but rather occurs in multiple limbs and may be subclinical.
- Once SLL is clinically apparent, lesions are usually well advanced, making recovery unlikely; therefore, the focus should be on prevention.
- Monitoring and enhancement of limb load cycling are key strategies for prevention of SLL.

INTRODUCTION

Laminitis is a well-recognized consequence of altered weight bearing due to pain or dysfunction in one or more limbs and, despite improvements in the management of catastrophic fractures and other complicated limb conditions, laminitis in the opposite ("supporting") limb remains a major cause of treatment failure in these cases. Compared with laminitis associated with hyperinsulinemia or sepsis, supporting limb laminitis (SLL) is less common and relatively poorly studied. In the last decade, there have been advances in the understanding of the pathogenesis of SLL. This new knowledge of key events may help to refine the management of clinical cases at risk and ultimately improve the ability to prevent SLL.

PREVALENCE, RISK FACTORS, AND CLINICAL PRESENTATION

Painful conditions that cause protracted alterations in weight bearing and ambulation, such as fractures and orthopedic infections, are considered to put horses at the

Department of Clinical Studies, New Bolton Center, School of Veterinary Medicine, University of Pennsylvania, 382 West Street Road, Kennett Square, PA 19348, USA
* Corresponding author.
E-mail address: vaneps@vet.upenn.edu

Vet Clin Equine 37 (2021) 657–668
https://doi.org/10.1016/j.cveq.2021.08.002

greatest risk of SLL.[1–3] In patient populations overall, the prevalence of SLL is low (0.02% in a recent study at a large UK hospital[4]); however, it is a relatively common complication in horses being treated for severe orthopedic problems. Of all horses that had a limb cast fitted over a 9-year period in one North American hospital, 12% developed SLL.[5] In another study examining cases where locking compression plate fixation was used for a variety of orthopedic conditions, 16% of all horses developed SLL and 25% of horses that specifically underwent fetlock arthrodeses were reportedly humanely euthanized owing to complications associated with SLL.[6] It is therefore evident that SLL is a significant cause of treatment failure in complex orthopedic cases. However, interpretation of the limited epidemiologic data available for SLL is problematic for 2 major reasons. First, the perceived risk of SLL in these cases is likely to be a barrier, which discourages even attempting treatment for certain orthopedic problems, which, in other species not prone to SLL, might be considered routine. This impact is not quantified in existing studies but warrants evaluation. Second, an accurate diagnosis of SLL is hampered in clinical cases by the presence of preexisting severe lameness in one or more limbs owing to the primary problem. As a result, SLL is often not clinically apparent until it has progressed sufficiently to cause lameness that exceeds that of the primarily injured limb, or until displacement of the distal phalanx within the hoof capsule is severe enough to cause appreciable clinical or radiographic changes.[7] It is therefore likely that SLL is more common than has been reported in these high-risk patient groups. Furthermore, it is unclear whether subclinical SLL may have an impact on recovery and return to athletic function in these cases. Although severe prolonged lameness is considered to predispose horses to the development of SLL, only the duration of lameness[2] (or duration of cast application[5]) and body weight[5] have been identified as significant risk factors. Furthermore, SLL can be difficult to predict from clinical assessments alone: some horses develop SLL despite apparently mild lameness, and others with severe lameness for prolonged periods do not. Accurate prediction and detection of SLL may require more sensitive and objective means of monitoring changes in limb weight-bearing patterns.

WHAT CAUSES SUPPORTING LIMB LAMINITIS AND HOW DOES IT DIFFER FROM OTHER FORMS OF LAMINITIS?

There is growing evidence that the 3 major "forms" of laminitis (sepsis-related, endocrine-associated, and SLL), although similar in terms of outcome (mechanical failure of the lamellae and a characteristic lameness), differ in terms of the primary mechanisms that lead to their development.[8] Ischemia has long been implicated as an underlying cause of SLL.[9–14] Studies using contrast radiography and computed tomography imaging[3,13] as well as Doppler ultrasound[14,15] have demonstrated that weight bearing affects perfusion in the major blood vessels of the foot. Furthermore, a study using near infrared spectroscopy (NIRS) showed an apparent effect (although variable) of short-term increased weight-bearing load on perfusion and oxygenation in the dorsal lamellar tissue.[16] More recently, the effects of longer-term, modest increases in weight-bearing load have been examined using a novel experimental preferential weight-bearing model. A nonpainful platform shoe insert was used to experimentally induce preferential weight bearing, resulting in extra load on the contralateral limb equivalent to approximately 10% of body weight (the equivalent of an extra 50 kg distributed onto a single limb in a 500-kg horse).[17] When preferential weight bearing was induced using this model for 48 hours in normal horses, it caused lamellar signaling changes (increased expression of hypoxia-inducible factor-1 alpha) suggestive of ischemia.[17] In a subsequent study, this same model was combined with tissue microdialysis, a technique that can detect temporal changes in lamellar perfusion and metabolism.[18] The prolonged, continuous increase in limb weight-bearing load was associated with evidence of ischemia (increased microdialysate lactate:pyruvate in particular). The ischemia became apparent after approximately 36 to 44 hours of preferential weight bearing and occurred specifically in the lamellar dermis; the adjacent sublamellar dermis (within the same foot) appeared unaffected. Ischemia was not detected in the absence of preferential limb load under otherwise identical conditions (confinement to stocks for a 92-hour experimental period). Similar microdialysis experiments failed to demonstrate lamellar ischemia in a model of acute sepsis-related laminitis[19] and during laminitis induction using hyperinsulinemia[20] (**Fig. 1**). Therefore, current evidence suggests that ischemia is important to the development of SLL, but not to the development of other forms of acute laminitis.

Because the maintenance of the lamellar cellular adhesions required to withstand mechanical stresses associated with weight bearing is an energy-consuming process, negative energy balance caused by reduced perfusion can rapidly affect the integrity of the lamellar tissue. Indeed, glucose deprivation in vitro causes disruption of lamellar adhesions and loss of lamellar structural integrity.[21,22] Cells furthest from the blood supply are likely to be preferentially affected by ischemia, and this is consistent with histologic findings in both the preferential weight-bearing model and natural SLL. Contrary to what is typical of acute laminitis owing to sepsis or hyperinsulinemia, evidence of cell death focused on the region immediately adjacent to the keratinized axes of the primary epidermal lamellae is a prominent feature in tissue from the preferential weight-bearing model (**Fig. 2**), and similarly, lesions in natural cases of SLL include cell death in this region (**Fig. 3**). It is also important to recognize that the lamellar lesions in SLL cases are not confined to the supporting limb (the limb contralateral to the primary injury). Instead, gross and histologic evidence of laminitis is commonly observed in multiple (and sometimes all) limbs of affected horses, including the primarily injured limb.[23,24] Furthermore, laminitis lesions in multiple limbs often vary in anatomic severity, and some may be subclinical.[23,24] Similarly, histologic lesions are identified in multiple limbs from horses in the preferential weight-bearing model (A.

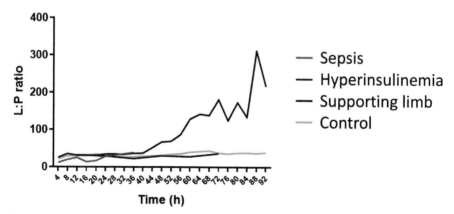

Fig. 1. Median tissue lactate-to-pyruvate ratio (L:P; a marker of ischemia) measured using lamellar tissue microdialysis in experimental models relevant to the 3 major forms of laminitis. The marked increase in L:P in the preferential weight-bearing model, but not in other models, demonstrates that ischemia is likely to be important in the pathogenesis of SLL, but not acute laminitis associated with sepsis or hyperinsulinemia.

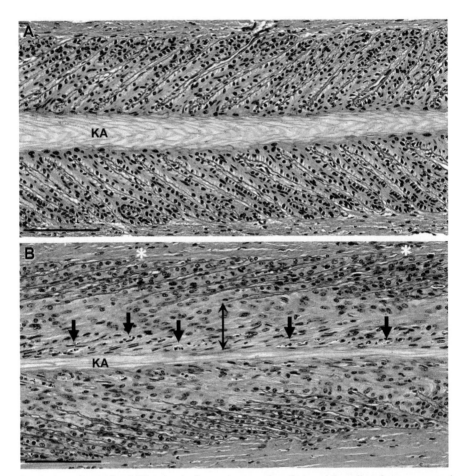

Fig. 2. Periodic acid Schiff-stained photomicrographs of dorsal lamellae from a normal horse (*A*) compared with one from an experimental preferential weight-bearing model (*B*). Some changes seen with preferential weight bearing are consistent with other forms of acute laminitis, including extensive elongation and thinning of secondary epidermal lamellae and detachment of basement membrane (*asterisks*). However, the presence of extensive cell death (pyknotic and karyorrhectic nuclei, *arrows*) adjacent to the keratinized axis (KA) is a unique finding. This is likely a consequence of poor perfusion and ischemia, which is more pronounced in this area, which is furthest from the blood supply. At approximately 2 days after metabolic evidence of ischemia (see **Fig. 1**), there is acanthosis of the parabasal cells with increased distance between the tips of the secondary dermal lamellae and KA (*double-headed arrow*), which may exacerbate the ischemic condition of these cells. Magnification = ×20. Bar = 200 μm.

van Eps, unpublished data, 2021). Current evidence therefore supports the theory that altered ambulation, rather than just increased limb load, interferes with normal lamellar microvascular perfusion, leading to negative energy balance and cellular dysfunction/death. This may be exacerbated by increased weight-bearing load, contributing to rapid and progressive failure of the lamellae and resultant acute laminitis that is most commonly evident in the supporting limb. A gradient of severity in terms of negative energy balance and cellular stress may contribute to a variety of dysfunctional

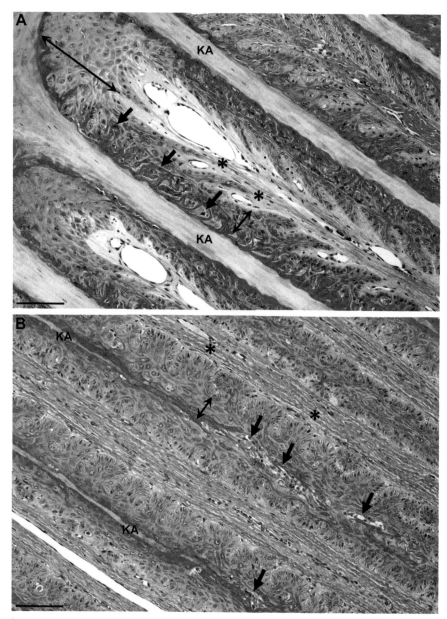

Fig. 3. Hematoxylin and eosin-stained photomicrographs of dorsal lamellae from a horse with naturally occurring acute SLL. (*A*) In abaxial regions of the primary epidermal lamellae, like the histology in the preferential weight-bearing model (see **Fig. 2**), some secondary epidermal lamellae demonstrate elongation and thinning (*asterisks*). Extensive cell death (cell shrinkage and hypereosinophilia with nuclear pyknosis and karyorrhexis; *arrows*) is concentrated in regions adjacent to the KA, and there is parabasal acanthosis (*double-headed arrows*). (*B*) In midregions of the primary epidermal lamellae, there is abaxial displacement of the KA that leaves linear clefts filled with fibrin, cell debris, and regenerating parabasal cells (*arrows*). Secondary epidermal lamellae are blunted with acanthosis of parabasal layers (*double-headed arrows*). Magnification = ×10. Bar = 100 μm.

processes within the lamellae across different limbs of the same patient that translate to various clinical and anatomic manifestations. Dysplasia of parabasal keratinocytes resulting in acanthosis with aberrant or accelerated cornification, triggered by hypoxia/reduced nutrient availability, appears to contribute to SLL, just as active cornification with widening of keratinized axes is a feature of naturally occurring endocrinopathic laminitis.[24,25] Upstream from keratinocyte death, cell stress pathways, including endoplasmic reticulum stress and the unfolded protein response (as demonstrated in endocrinopathic laminitis[25]), may be induced by hypoxia and low nutrient availability in SLL, contributing to keratinocyte dysfunction and weakening of the lamellae. Apart from negative energy balance and ischemia, it is likely that other mechanisms may also contribute to the development of SLL. Activation of the interleukin-17 (IL-17)-dependent inflammatory pathway is an epidermal stress response that contributes to skin diseases, such as psoriasis,[26] and could contribute to many of the events central to laminitis progression, including adhesion loss, stretch, and altered cellular differentiation. Recently, upregulation of several IL-17 target genes has been demonstrated in natural cases of SLL.[23] Consistent, abnormal increases in limb load may also affect mechanical stresses in the lamellae sufficiently to alter mechanostasis, triggering cell death and proliferative responses and subsequent remodeling of the tissue.[27] There is evidence that remodeling occurs within the lamellae in response to normal mechanical stresses associated with locomotion,[28–31] and the effects of abnormal mechanical stresses on these events warrant study. Systemic disease or dysfunction may also contribute to the development of SLL. Systemic inflammation can be present in horses at risk of SLL, particularly when infection is a component of the primary limb condition.[23] In addition, it is likely that insulin dysregulation may also be present in some horses at risk of developing SLL, and severe pain is known to exacerbate this. The association between these systemic factors and the development of SLL has not been studied and needs investigation.

WHAT STRATEGIES CAN BE USED TO PREVENT SUPPORTING LIMB LAMINITIS?

In the authors' experience, there is no shoe, orthotic manipulation, or stall surface that can prevent the development of SLL, and there are no published controlled studies demonstrating the efficacy of any preventative measure. Based on current evidence, the areas of focus to advance toward effective means of preventing SLL in the future should be (1) to develop and deploy means of accurately characterizing and monitoring ambulatory and weight-bearing patterns in horses at risk of SLL in the clinic; and (2) to target therapy that specifically supports ambulatory activity or promotes limb load cycling in cases whereby ambulation is not possible owing to pain or dysfunction.

Microdialysis studies demonstrate that lamellar microvascular perfusion is dependent on cyclic limb load and apparently cannot be enhanced in the static horse using drugs or orthotic manipulations.[32,33] This is consistent with observations made in a cadaver limb model,[34] where consistent fill of lamellar dermal microvasculature only occurred when arterial perfusion was coupled with cyclic vertical load (**Fig. 4**). It follows that those strategies to monitor and enhance limb load cycling are likely to be the key to improving lamellar perfusion and preventing SLL. Monitoring should include some form of continuous quantification of limb load cycling activity, preferably for individual limbs. Systems validated for monitoring locomotor activity and step counts in horses have been described.[35,36] A method that can detect not only walking steps but also more subtle weight-shifting events in individual limbs requires development and validation; however, preliminary testing of a hoof mounted accelerometer system

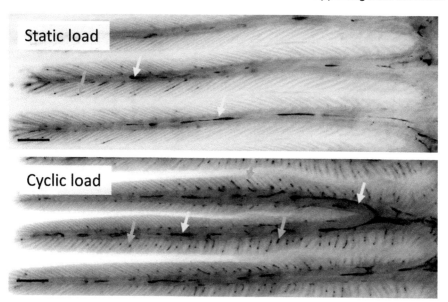

Fig. 4. Photomicrographs of unstained middorsal lamellar sections from cadaver forelimbs from the same horse, arterially perfused with a marker solution while subjected to either static vertical load (*top*) or cyclic vertical load (*bottom*) equivalent to 30% bwt. The perfusion marker (*black*) is visible in primary dermal lamellar vasculature (*yellow arrows*) and secondary dermal lamellar capillaries (*blue arrows*). Cyclic load was necessary for consistent SDL capillary fill in this model, in agreement with the observation in live horse microdialysis studies that lamellar perfusion is dependent on cyclic limb load (ambulation as well as limb weight shifting when at rest). Unstained sections, ×10 magnification. Bar = 200 μm. bwt, bodyweight.

(**Fig. 5**) suggests that monitoring the frequency of these offloading events may be a useful means of identifying SLL risk (associated with reduced weight-shifting frequency) and also a novel means of early acute SLL detection (associated with increased weight-shifting frequency). To enhance load cycling, regular encouragement to walk may be beneficial; however, there are currently insufficient data to support specific recommendations, and, in some horses, walking may not be achievable because of the nature of the primary limb condition. The development of novel dynamic sling technology allows for dynamic, partial, or total load reduction on one or multiple limbs, and this may improve management in these cases.[37] Provision of multimodal analgesia, particularly using regional techniques,[38] may help to normalize limb weight distribution and cycling frequency in horses at risk of SLL; however, medications with a sedative effect may be best avoided because they may reduce voluntary ambulation and limb load cycling.

Development of practical techniques to monitor the metabolic health of the lamellar tissue itself in clinical patients may be critical for successful prevention and management of SLL. Although microdialysis is used clinically for monitoring cerebral metabolism in human patients with brain injury[39] and has been used extensively in equine laminitis research, it is expensive and not practical for long-term monitoring in the horse foot. The other disadvantage of probe-based monitoring methods, including microdialysis and NIRS, is that sampling is confined to 1 area, whereas laminitis development and the distribution of pathologic lesions is often regional and heterogeneous. Recently, the use of PET with ^{18}F-fluorodeoxyglucose has been described in the equine distal limb.[40] An advantage of PET is that changes in tissue

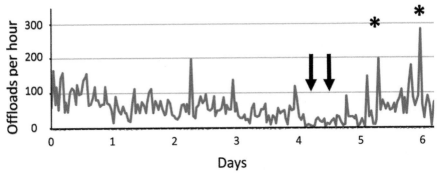

Fig. 5. Limb motion activity in the contralateral limb of a horse hospitalized for treatment of a fracture. The frequency of steps and standing weight-shifting episodes ("offloads") per hour was determined using a custom hoof mounted accelerometer device and bespoke machine learning algorithm. The frequency of offloads decreases over several days of hospitalization, reaching a minimum (*arrows*) before a sudden increase in weight-shifting frequency (*asterisks*), which coincided with the clinical recognition and radiographic diagnosis of SLL in this case. Studies are needed to confirm whether reduced ambulatory activity and limb offloading frequency are associated with the development of SLL. This type of monitoring may be useful in clinical patients for early identification of SLL risk and to guide potential intervention.

metabolism (glucose tracer uptake) can be detected and localized using high-resolution 3-dimensional images of the entire foot. The technique is possible in the standing horse with current equipment, and therefore, PET may be a clinically useful means of monitoring global lamellar health in horses at risk of SLL.

CLINICAL SIGNS, DIAGNOSIS, AND MANAGEMENT OF SUPPORTING LIMB LAMINITIS

The clinical presentation of SLL is like that of other forms of laminitis; however, the lameness is often masked by that of the primary limb problem. Furthermore, severe preexisting lameness hampers efforts to conduct a conventional thorough physical examination. The most obvious clinical indicator for SLL is a sudden apparent improvement in lameness in the limb with the primary condition (owing to the development of lameness in the supporting limb). In these cases, more frequent weight shifting off the supporting limb may also be evident. An increase in heart rate is often seen as an early indicator of SLL, and the change may be subtle, highlighting the usefulness of serial or continuous measurements. On examination of the supporting limb, there may be an increase in digital pulse amplitude and consistent warmth of the dorsal hoof wall, although these findings are inconsistent and inconclusive alone or in combination. An increased prominence of the coronary band may be an early indicator of displacement of the distal phalanx, and this may progress to a palpable "cleft" at the coronary band. Hoof testing is unreliable and often difficult to perform in these cases because of preexisting lameness. Radiographic imaging can be used to detect changes in the position of the distal phalanx relative to the hoof wall. The earliest changes are seen in the coronary band-extensor process distance ("founder distance") and the dorsal hoof wall-distal phalanx distance, both of which may be measured on a lateral-medial radiograph (**Fig. 6**). With high-quality radiographs, it is possible to measure the thickness of the more radiolucent portion of the dorsal hoof wall region, which is not affected by hoof wall trimming and may more accurately reflect dimensional changes

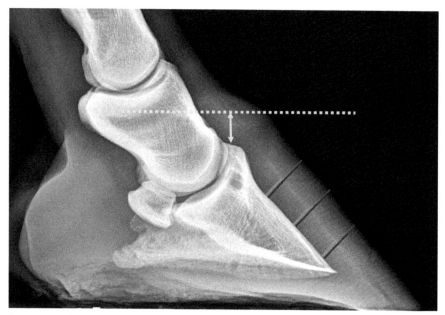

Fig. 6. Lateral-to-medial radiograph of a normal foot demonstrating measurement techniques that are most useful for monitoring in horses at risk of SLL. The distance from extensor process to coronary band (*yellow;* using a dotted guideline parallel to ground surface) is an indicator of distal displacement of the coronary band. This measurement varies between horses and between feet, but normal values are reported to be approximately 6.5 to 7.5 mm. Dorsal hoof wall to distal phalanx distance (*purple lines*) can also vary but usually does not exceed approximately18 mm in clinically normal horses. Measurement of the thickness of the more radiolucent area of the dorsal hoof wall (*blue lines*) may be performed on most digital radiographs and may be a more sensitive method of detecting physical changes specific to the lamellae. The normal thickness of this layer is approximately 7 to 8 mm or less in normal horses. All measurements are best performed serially to detect subtle changes over time in horses at risk of SLL.

in the lamellae.[41] There is often minimal or no change in the angle between dorsal hoof wall and distal phalanx in SLL cases.[2] Serial radiographs with measurements, beginning at presentation and repeated as often as weekly, increase the probability of early detection of SLL.

Once a diagnosis is made, recommendations for the management of SLL are like that of acute laminitis due to other causes and include provision for frog and caudal sole support through application of shoes or orthotics and ensuring adequate analgesia. In acute cases with rapid progression, the prognosis is considered poor, particularly if the primary limb condition is unresolved.

SUMMARY

Although SLL continues to impact the ability to successfully manage horses with painful limb conditions, recent improvements in the understanding of why laminitis occurs in these cases is paving the way for strategies to help prevent it. New evidence confirms that ischemia, owing to a lack of normal cyclic limb load, leads to cell dysfunction and death within the lamellae and that this is not confined to the contralateral (supporting) limb alone. Progression to acute laminitis in the supporting limb is enhanced by excessive load and can be rapid and severe. Current evidence suggests that prevention of SLL will rely on the development and clinical utilization of systems to monitor and safely encourage cyclic limb load in horses with painful limb injuries.

ACKNOWLEDGEMENTS

The presented work is supported by grants from the Grayson Jockey Club Research Foundation. Grant IDs (GJCRF identifies by title only, there is no number). Laminar Signaling in Supporting Limb Laminitis; Lamellar Energy Failure in Supporting Limb Laminitis; Weight Bearing; Perfusion and Bioenergetics in Laminitis; Prevention of Supporting Limb Laminitis.

DISCLOSURE

Nothing to disclose.

REFERENCES

1. Baxter GM, Morrison S. Complications of unilateral weight bearing. Vet Clin North Am Equine Pract 2008;24:621–42, ix.
2. Peloso JG, Cohen ND, Walker MA, et al. Case-control study of risk factors for the development of laminitis in the contralateral limb in Equidae with unilateral lameness. J Am Vet Med Assoc 1996;209:1746–9.
3. van Eps A, Collins SN, Pollitt CC. Supporting limb laminitis. Vet Clin North Am Equine Pract 2010;26:287–302.
4. Wylie CE, Newton JR, Bathe AP, et al. Prevalence of supporting limb laminitis in a UK equine practice and referral hospital setting between 2005 and 2013: implications for future epidemiological studies. Vet Rec 2015;176:72.
5. Virgin JE, Goodrich LR, Baxter GM, et al. Incidence of support limb laminitis in horses treated with half limb, full limb or transfixation pin casts: a retrospective study of 113 horses (2000-2009). Equine Vet J Suppl 2011;7–11.
6. Levine DG, Richardson DW. Clinical use of the locking compression plate (LCP) in horses: a retrospective study of 31 cases (2004-2006). Equine Vet J 2007;39: 401–6.
7. Baxter GM. Supporting limb laminitis. Hoboken (NJ): John Wiley and Sons, Inc.; 2017. p. 210–3.
8. van Eps AW, Burns TA. Are there shared mechanisms in the pathophysiology of different clinical forms of laminitis and what are the implications for prevention and treatment? Vet Clin North Am Equine Pract 2019;35:379–98.
9. Redden RF. Preventing laminitis in the contralateral limb of horses with non-weightbearing lameness. Clin Tech Equine Pract 2004;3:57–63.
10. Hood DM, Grosenbaugh DA, Mostafa MB, et al. The role of vascular mechanisms in the development of acute equine laminitis. J Vet Intern Med 1993;7:228–34.
11. Hood DM. The mechanisms and consequences of structural failure of the foot. Vet Clin North Am Equine Pract 1999;15:437–61.
12. Hood DM. The pathophysiology of developmental and acute laminitis. Vet Clin North Am Equine Pract 1999;15:321–43.
13. van Kraayenburg FJ, Fairall N, Littlejohn A: The effect of vertical force on blood flow in the palmar arteries of the horse. In 1st international congress on equine exercise physiology, Cambridge, pp 144-54.

14. Hoffmann KL, Wood AK, Griffiths KA, et al. Doppler sonographic measurements of arterial blood flow and their repeatability in the equine foot during weight bearing and non-weight bearing. Res Vet Sci 2001;70:199–203.

15. Pietra M, Guglielmini C, Nardi S, et al. Influence of weight bearing and hoof position on Doppler evaluation of lateral palmar digital arteries in healthy horses. Am J Vet Res 2004;65:1211–5.

16. Hinckley KA, Fearn S, Howard BR, et al. Near infrared spectroscopy of pedal haemodynamics and oxygenation in normal and laminitic horses. Equine Vet J 1995;27:465–70.

17. Gardner AK, van Eps AW, Watts MR, et al. A novel model to assess lamellar signaling relevant to preferential weight bearing in the horse. Vet J 2017; 221:62–7.

18. van Eps AW, Belknap JK, Schneider X, et al. Lamellar perfusion and energy metabolism in a preferential weight bearing model. Equine Vet J 2021;53:834–44.

19. Medina-Torres CE, Underwood C, Pollitt CC, et al. Microdialysis measurements of lamellar perfusion and energy metabolism during the development of laminitis in the oligofructose model. Equine Vet J 2016;48:246–52.

20. Stokes SM, Bertin FR, Stefanovski D, et al. The effect of continuous digital hypothermia on lamellar energy metabolism and perfusion during laminitis development in two experimental models. Equine Vet J 2020;52:585–92.

21. Pass MA, Pollitt S, Pollitt CC. Decreased glucose metabolism causes separation of hoof lamellae in vitro: a trigger for laminitis? Equine Vet J Suppl 1998;(26): 133–8.

22. French KR, Pollitt CC. Equine laminitis: glucose deprivation and MMP activation induce dermo-epidermal separation in vitro. Equine Vet J 2004;36:261–6.

23. Cassimeris L, Engiles JB, Galantino-Homer H. Interleukin-17A pathway target genes are upregulated in Equus caballus supporting limb laminitis. PLoS One 2020;15:e0232920.

24. Engiles JB, Galantino-Homer HL, Boston R, et al. Osteopathology in the equine distal phalanx associated with the development and progression of laminitis. Vet Pathol 2015;52:928–44.

25. Cassimeris L, Engiles JB, Galantino-Homer H. Detection of endoplasmic reticulum stress and the unfolded protein response in naturally-occurring endocrinopathic equine laminitis. BMC Vet Res 2019;15:24.

26. Prinz I, Sandrock I, Mrowietz U. Interleukin-17 cytokines: effectors and targets in psoriasis-a breakthrough in understanding and treatment. J Exp Med 2020;217: e20191397.

27. Chan DD, Van Dyke WS, Bahls M, et al. Mechanostasis in apoptosis and medicine. Prog Biophys Mol Biol 2011;106:517–24.

28. Thomason JJ, McClinchey HL, Faramarzi B, et al. Mechanical behavior and quantitative morphology of the equine laminar junction. Anat Rec A Discov Mol Cell Evol Biol 2005;283:366–79.

29. Thomason JJ, Faramarzi B, Revill A, et al. Quantitative morphology of the equine laminar junction in relation to capsule shape in the forehoof of standardbreds and thoroughbreds. Equine Vet J 2008;40:473–80.

30. Lancaster LS, Bowker RM, Mauer WA. Density and morphologic features of primary epidermal laminae in the feet of three-year-old racing quarter horses. Am J Vet Res 2007;68:11–9.

31. Faramarzi B. Morphological spectrum of primary epidermal laminae in the forehoof of thoroughbred horses. Equine Vet J 2011;43:732–6.

32. Medina-Torres CE, Underwood C, Pollitt CC, et al. Microdialysis measurements of equine lamellar perfusion and energy metabolism in response to physical and pharmacological manipulations of blood flow. Equine Vet J 2016;48:756–64.

33. Medina-Torres CE, Underwood C, Pollitt CC, et al. The effect of weightbearing and limb load cycling on equine lamellar perfusion and energy metabolism measured using tissue microdialysis. Equine Vet J 2016;48:114–9.

34. Ford MG, Torcivia C, Kowalski A, et al. The effect of mechanical load on lamellar microvascular perfusion in an equine cadaver limb model. In: American College of Veterinary Surgeons Summit, Virtual 2020;33.

35. Steinke SL, Montgomery JB, Barden JM. Accelerometry-based step count validation for horse movement analysis during stall confinement. Front Vet Sci 2021;8: 681213.

36. Maisonpierre IN, Sutton MA, Harris P, et al. Accelerometer activity tracking in horses and the effect of pasture management on time budget. Equine Vet J 2019;51:840–5.

37. Steinke SL, Carmalt JL, Montgomery B. Weight reduction and possible implications for the rehabilitation of horses with ambulatory difficulties. Equine Vet Educ 2019;33:152–8.

38. Hopster K, van Eps AW. Pain management for laminitis in the horse. Equine Vet Educ 2019;31:384–92.

39. Carteron L, Bouzat P, Oddo M. Cerebral microdialysis monitoring to improve individualized neurointensive care therapy: an update of recent clinical data. Front Neurol 2017;8:601.

40. Spriet M, Espinosa P, Kyme AZ, et al. Positron emission tomography of the equine distal limb: exploratory study. Vet Radiol Ultrasound 2016;57:630–8.

41. Grundmann IN, Drost WT, Zekas LJ, et al. Quantitative assessment of the equine hoof using digital radiography and magnetic resonance imaging. Equine Vet J 2015;47:542–7.

"Feeding the Foot"
Nutritional Influences on Equine Hoof Health

Teresa A. Burns, DVM, PhD

KEYWORDS

- Insulin dysregulation • Laminitis • Podiatry • Nutrition • Obesity
- Equine metabolic syndrome

KEY POINTS

- A balanced diet is essential for optimum growth and health of the entire horse, including the foot.
- The structures of the equine foot can be affected by conditions of nutritional excess (such as equine insulin dysregulation and equine metabolic syndrome, enteral carbohydrate overload, and selenosis) and nutritional deficiency (eg, zinc).
- Supplementation with vitamins, amino acids, and trace minerals that affect hoof growth and hoof horn quality may benefit horses who have clinical problems related to these characteristics.
- However, evidence to guide clinical practice in this area is lacking.
- An equine nutritionist should be consulted when creating a nutrition plan appropriate for the life stage, work level, and disease status of a particular equine patient.

INTRODUCTION

Nutrition is a highly influential factor governing the incidence, progression, and prognosis associated with many important diseases of humans and animals, particularly chronic conditions that result from nutritional excess (eg, type 2 diabetes mellitus, coronary artery disease, equine metabolic syndrome [EMS]). In fact, the pathophysiology of one of the most important diseases of the equine foot—laminitis—is directly linked to nutritional influences via multiple mechanisms, some of which are detailed elsewhere.[1] In this review, several significant nutritional influences on the health of the equine foot will be described. Although this description will not be a comprehensive review of any facet of equine nutrition *per se*, interested readers can access additional information in other excellent reviews published on the topic.[2–8] In this review, selected macronutrients and micronutrients of interest to the health of the equine foot are discussed.

Department of Veterinary Clinical Sciences, The Ohio State University, Columbus, OH, USA
E-mail address: burns.402@osu.edu

Vet Clin Equine 37 (2021) 669–684
https://doi.org/10.1016/j.cveq.2021.07.004
0749-0739/21/© 2021 Elsevier Inc. All rights reserved.

vetequine.theclinics.com

MACRONUTRIENTS
Dietary Carbohydrate

By far, the vast majority of research and clinical interest regarding the influence of nutrition on the health of the equine foot has centered on dietary carbohydrate content, particularly that fraction that is most likely to affect postprandial blood glucose concentrations and, therefore, the capacity to promote hyperinsulinemia. Hyperinsulinemia is now well-established as one of the most important risk factors for the development of endocrinopathic laminitis, whether it be related to EMS, pituitary pars intermedia dysfunction, iatrogenic corticosteroid administration, or some other condition associated with insulin dysregulation (ID). Several groups have identified this link independently in cross-sectional and prospective observational studies of equine populations, where the presence and degree of hyperinsulinemia were both associated with the development of laminitis.[9–11] A more direct link between hyperinsulinemia and laminitis has been established through the experimental induction of laminitis via iatrogenic hyperinsulinemia in normal ponies and, subsequently, normal light breed horses.[12,13] Insulin is a pleiotropic hormone whose functions are not limited to regulation of carbohydrate, lipid, and protein metabolism in the postprandial period (even though this is where most attention has been directed). Insulin signaling through its own receptor, through insulin-like growth factor-1 receptor (IGF1-R), or hybrids of these 2 receptors has been shown to activate not only pathways that direct the fates of nutritional metabolites (through PI3K activation), but also the modulation of cellular proliferation and metabolism of components of the extracellular matrix (through the activation of mitogen-activated protein kinase pathways).[14] These mechanisms could clearly relate to the digital lamellar lesions that develop in the presence of hyperinsulinemia (keratinocyte proliferation, lamellar stretching, and detachment of lamellar basal epithelial cells from their basement membrane).[15–17] Given that very little insulin receptor is expressed by lamellar keratinocytes, a direct effect of insulin on these cells is most likely mediated through the IGF-1R[18,19]; recent in vitro and in vivo studies have supported this explanation,[20,21] including evidence that the administration of an equinized human anti–IGF-1R monoclonal antibody can attenuate the lamellar lesion induced by experimental hyperinsulinemia.[22] Although the precise molecular mechanisms involved require further clarification, given the strong association of hyperinsulinemia with endocrinopathic laminitis, nutritional interventions should be directed toward minimizing postprandial insulin secretion and maximizing systemic insulin sensitivity. Some techniques for nutritional management of horses with ID are described later in this article.

It is important to bear in mind that during the euglycemic–hyperinsulinemic clamp method for experimental induction of endocrinopathic laminitis, insulin is not the only experimental variable; glucose is continuously infused along with insulin to maintain euglycemia in the face of profound hyperinsulinemia. This consideration is important, given that the bulk of glucose uptake by keratinocytes of the digital lamellae is most likely to be continuous and passive down its concentration gradient through glucose transporters that are not insulin dependent. Previous work has demonstrated that the digital lamellae have a relatively high metabolic demand for glucose[23] and that lamellar keratinocytes express primarily glucose transporter 1 (GLUT1; a noninsulin responsive glucose transporter) to accommodate this substrate demand.[24] Interestingly, under conditions of the EHC, where GLUT1 transporter expression is actively down-regulated in tissues that are insulin-dependent (such as skeletal muscle), digital lamellar GLUT1 expression is unchanged, theoretically allowing for increased lamellar glucose uptake under these conditions.[25] Exposure to glucose alone is sufficient to activate signaling pathways commonly associated with insulin and IGF-1 receptor activation in cultured equine keratinocytes,[26] and glucose alone can drive epithelial cells through epithelial-to-mesenchymal transition (a process that has been associated with equine laminitis).[27–30] It is also reasonable to assume that glucose exposure is increased in the digital lamellae of equids with ID, particularly after the ingestion of feedstuffs containing high concentrations of nonstructural carbohydrates (**Fig. 1**). Therefore, minimizing postprandial hyperglycemia in horses with ID is important not only because this practice can minimize hyperinsulinemia, but also to minimize the potential deleterious effects of glucose itself on the digital lamellae.

Before discussing dietary modifications further, a brief comment defining the relevant carbohydrate fractions included in a proximate analysis of feedstuffs may be helpful. Nonstructural carbohydrate is the term often used to refer to those components of the carbohydrate fraction originating from plant cell contents (in contrast with those originating from plant cell walls, which make up the neutral detergent fiber). The nonstructural carbohydrates include those carbohydrates most likely to influence postprandial insulin and glucose dynamics, and this is the fraction of the diet that has been the target of most dietary composition interventions for patients with EMS. Nonstructural carbohydrate is a measure of hydrolyzable carbohydrate, encompassing simple sugars, disaccharides, oligosaccharides, fructans, and starches. Ethanol-soluble carbohydrate represents simple sugars, disaccharides, and oligosaccharides, and water-soluble carbohydrate represents ethanol-soluble carbohydrate and fructans.[31] Nonstructural carbohydrates can therefore be represented in the following ways:

1. Simple sugars + disaccharides + oligosaccharides + fructans + starches
2. Ethanol-soluble carbohydrate + fructans + starches
3. Water-soluble carbohydrate + starches

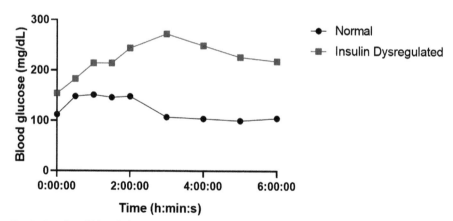

Fig. 1. Results of blood glucose concentration measurements during an oral sugar test in the same horse before (normal) and after (insulin dysregulated) induction of ID with dexamethasone (0.08 mg/kg by mouth once per day for 7 days). The baseline blood glucose concentration is higher in association with ID, as is the area under the blood glucose-time curve in response to an enteral carbohydrate challenge. Digital lamellar glucose exposure after high-carbohydrate feeding will be higher in ID individuals than in animals with normal insulin and glucose dynamics.

The dietary management of horses and ponies with ID involves 3 general approaches, all aimed at minimizing the duration and magnitude of hyperinsulinemia:

1. Reduction of the nonstructural carbohydrate content of the diet (all components)

   Although blood glucose is not the only secretagogue for insulin, it is by far the most important, and dietary nonstructural carbohydrate content is positively correlated with postprandial blood glucose (and insulin) concentrations in horses.

2. Limiting the size of meals and rate of ingestion of feedstuffs

   As for the comments about composition discussed elsewhere in this article, this also applies to all components of the diet but is particularly relevant to pasture. Pasture access represents a relatively uncontrolled and poorly quantifiable source of dietary intake generally (and nonstructural carbohydrate content, specifically); therefore, removing a horse from pasture until ID is improved is appropriate.

3. General caloric restriction until ideal body weight has been achieved (if weight loss is indicated)

   Obesity is associated with ID (particularly systemic and tissue insulin resistance) in many species, including horses, and insulin and glucose dynamics are often improved after weight loss. ID may persist after weight loss in individuals of breeds and types that are predisposed to EMS, and management of the composition of the diet (more so than caloric restriction *per se*) will remain important for these horses long-term, even if relatively lean.

The first approach intuitively involves removal of cereal grains and other concentrate feeds from the horse's diet and the selection of forage with a relatively low nonstructural carbohydrate content, which can be determined by submitting a sample for proximate analysis. Recommendations frequently state that the nonstructural carbohydrate content of the diet should ideally fall below 10% on a dry matter basis in all dietary components, and indeed, studies using diets with this composition show improved insulin and glucose dynamics in horses consuming them when compared with more conventional equine diets.[32–35] However, this number has not been subjected to critical scrutiny, and this recommendation may well change in response to future investigations. The relative importance of nonstructural carbohydrate intake also likely varies with the severity of ID. Horses with severe ID (resting insulin concentration of >100 μIU/mL) may do best when maintained on a stringent diet with an nonstructural carbohydrate content of less than 10%, whereas mildly affected horses can likely be fed diets with slightly higher nonstructural carbohydrate contents (cautiously). If the nonstructural carbohydrate content of a particular hay is greater than 10%, soaking may be a way to render it safer for feeding to horses with ID. Protocols utilizing soaking alone (16 °C for 9 hours), steaming (50 minutes in a hay steamer) followed by soaking, or soaking followed by steaming all seem to be equally effective at decreasing the nonstructural carbohydrate content of hay (approximately 30%), with soaking followed by steaming resulting in the lowest levels of microbial contamination within the final product.[36] Soaked hay has been shown to induce lower postprandial insulinemic responses in ponies compared with those fed dry hay or haylage,[37] and feeding soaked hay has been associated with accelerated weight loss in overweight horses and ponies.[38] Using warmer soaking water can result in more effective nonstructural carbohydrate leaching from forage, but this practice also accelerates microbial proliferation within the product, may cause hygienic concerns with feeding,[39–41] and may render the forage less palatable to some horses.[42] Other strategies for decreasing the nonstructural carbohydrate content of pasture have been reviewed previously.[5,6,43]

The second approach, limiting or slowing the rate of ingestion of feedstuffs, can be accomplished in several ways, many of which have been objectively demonstrated to influence the amount of consumption and, in some cases, postprandial insulin and glucose dynamics in horses and ponies. Grazing muzzles can effectively control the rate of weight gain in ponies at pasture when worn for 10 hours per day, but significant individual variability exists with respect to response to this treatment.[44] When ponies were required to walk additional distance to access feed from a customized, timed feeder, researchers reported lower body condition scores in association with this practice (but no significant change in insulin and glucose dynamics).[45] In another study, the addition of a relatively small amount of daily exercise (15 minutes of trot) to dietary restrictions resulted in more tangible improvements in hormonal variables in the absence of weight loss.[46] Limiting the feeding of forage using a slow feed hay net has been shown to extend the time to meal consumption and delay peak postprandial insulin concentration in overweight light breed horses.[47] Finally, strip grazing practices have been shown to result in lower dry matter consumption and gains in body weight in ponies compared with free access to a total pasture area.[48] Most of these techniques are accessible and feasible and can improve the nutritional management of horses and ponies with ID.

The third approach, caloric restriction until an appropriate body condition has been achieved, is appropriate for most patients with EMS (at least initially). Weight loss should be encouraged in overweight or obese horses by decreasing the total number of daily calories consumed. In horses that are overweight and being overfed (which is often the case), removing all concentrate feed(s) from the diet can be enough to allow the horse to achieve its ideal body weight within 8 to 12 weeks. Total caloric intake should initially be met by feeding hay (ideally a grass hay tested and determined to contain <10% nonstructural carbohydrate) in amounts equivalent to 1.5% to 2.0% of current body weight. If the horse does not lose weight as expected over 6 to 8 weeks, the amount fed can be decreased gradually over several weeks to 1.0% to 1.5% of ideal body weight.[49,50] Feeding less than 1.0% of ideal body weight in forage per day is not recommended, because this amount may represent an unsafe risk of hyperlipidemia and hyperlipemia in overweight equids with ID.[51–53]

These strategies are effective for horses kept in stalls or dirt paddocks, but weight loss can be more difficult to achieve when horses are grazing on pasture (because this practice represents a dietary component whose consumption is difficult to quantify or control effectively). Strategies for limiting grass consumption on pasture include restricted (eg, <1 hour) turnout periods; confinement to a small paddock, round pen, or area enclosed with moveable tape/fencing (see comments regarding strip grazing elsewhere in this article); or the use of a grazing muzzle. Appropriate vitamin and mineral supplements should be provided to horses confined to dirt paddocks or stalls or whose daily forage ration consists of a restricted amount of grass hay. Pasture access should remain restricted until measures of insulin and glucose dynamics have improved, because the nonstructural carbohydrates consumed on pasture can trigger laminitis rapidly in susceptible horses.

Horses with recurrent laminitis may require housing away from pasture indefinitely. These animals should be housed in dirt paddocks so that they are able to move freely and exercise once laminitis has been controlled. Mildly affected horses can be returned to pasture if ID can be managed, but care should be taken to restrict pasture access when the grass is going through dynamic phases, such as rapid growth in the spring or the onset of cold weather in the fall. The measurement of the nonstructural carbohydrate content of pasture grass at different times of the day has revealed that grazing in the early morning is likely to be safer for horses with ID, except after a hard frost when grasses often accumulate sugars and fructans.

Lean horses with ID are challenging to manage from a nutritional standpoint, because additional calories must be provided without exacerbating ID. This goal can usually be accomplished by feeding one of the low-sugar/low-starch (low-nonstructural carbohydrate) pelleted feeds that are now available commercially. These feeds vary in their nonstructural carbohydrate content, so that value should be determined and the severity of ID taken into account before one is selected. Dividing the daily ration into multiple small meals and feeding hay before concentrate can also help to blunt the postprandial blood glucose curve when feeding concentrate products.[6] Individual horses may respond differently to the same feed, so it is advisable to monitor insulin and glucose dynamics regularly, including (ideally) 7 to 14 days after a new diet has been initiated. Severely ID horses can be particularly difficult to manage and would benefit from individual diet formulation with the help of an equine nutritionist, particularly as recommendations become more restrictive. Rinsed and soaked molasses-free beet pulp can be fed as a more economical alternative to commercial feeds.[54,55] This feedstuff induces a low glycemic response, yet provides calories through hindgut fermentation and volatile fatty acid production. Fat and fiber are safer sources of calories than nonstructural carbohydrate for ID horses that need to maintain or gain weight.[34,56,57]

Dietary Fat

Although dietary fat is often used to increase the energy density of equine rations for the purpose of improving body condition (or maintaining it in the face of increased caloric requirements, such as with intense exercise or late-term gestation or lactation), this specific macronutrient is not known to have a measurable effect on the rate of hoof growth or hoof quality (although at least 1 study has demonstrated the possibility of modifying the lipid composition of the hoof wall with supplementation, in this case with evening primrose oil[58]). Dietary fat should be leveraged to treat horses at risk of suffering adverse effects on hoof quality associated with starvation or chronic protein–calorie malnutrition, which are more clearly established. Adult horses can tolerate a diet relatively high in fat (15%–20% of digestible energy[59]) if the transition to this level of supplementation is made gradually over a period of 10 to 14 days.

Dietary Protein

The effects of dietary protein deficiency are generally nonspecific and may also be related to the accompanying caloric restriction (protein–calorie malnutrition). Veterinarians will likely recognize that poor quality hair coat and poor hoof growth (including abnormal growth rings) are common in affected horses; these conditions usually improve over time with normalization of the diet, but permanent injury can be incurred with severe protein restriction of young, growing animals. Relatively little attention has been given to the role of dietary protein and amino acids in the health of the foot, although certain sulfur-containing amino acids, such as cysteine and methionine, are known to be important structural components of keratinized tissue and are rapidly taken up by lamellar keratinocytes after local infusion into digital vessels.[60] Other amino acids, notably lysine and threonine, are reported to be those most limiting in the equine diet, and most nutritional recommendations for horses are formed around them to some degree.[61] Many equine hoof supplements currently on the market contain specific amino acids to support keratin production and improved hoof quality (cysteine, methionine, lysine, proline, and tyrosine are common), but little evidence is available currently to support specific outcomes resulting from this practice.

The vast majority of recent investigations into nutritional influences on the equine foot have been related to dietary nonstructural carbohydrate content, ID, and endocrinopathic laminitis (as discussed elsewhere in this article); in comparison, very little is known about the relevance of dietary protein and amino acid composition to these processes. In fact, that influence has been broadly assumed to be minimal, given the frequency with which ration balancers that contain vitamins, trace minerals, and a relatively high protein content (typically in the 32%–35% dry matter range) are recommended to accompany the low nonstructural carbohydrate grass hay that composes the bulk of the diet of equids with ID.[49] These products are not fed in great quantity (typically 1–3 pounds per 500 kg horse per day), although their protein content is such that postprandial increases in plasma amino acid concentrations could be anticipated. Although blood glucose is the most important, physiologically relevant stimulus for insulin secretion in the postprandial period (making it a rational target for dietary interventions to control hyperinsulinemia), it is not the only one; certain amino acids (notably arginine) are also known to induce insulin secretion when their plasma concentrations increase.[62–64] This effect has been assumed to have a minor contributory role to postprandial insulin secretion in horses, but some recent evidence suggests that dietary protein content and relative amino acid abundance can influence postprandial insulin secretion in a way that may be highly relevant to management of equine ID.[65] In a study comparing horses with EMS (n = 6) with unaffected controls, a high protein meal (similar in composition to that found in many ration balancer products, albeit fed at approximately twice the recommended daily rate) was associated with a 9-fold increase in postprandial insulin secretion in horses with EMS compared with control horses; blood glucose concentrations were not different between the 2 groups.[65] These data strongly suggest that additional investigation of dietary protein and its effects on equine hyperinsulinemia is needed to optimize dietary recommendations for patients with EMS, because high protein feedstuffs are included in these recommendations currently.[49] It is also important to bear in mind that even though dietary protein may adversely affect insulin and glucose dynamics in EMS, individual amino acids may be beneficial in this setting; for example, feeding a supplement containing a proprietary combination of leucine and resveratrol was associated with decreased insulin responses to an oral sugar test in horses with ID.[66] Additional work is needed to provide guidance for veterinarians and horse owners caring for these animals.

MICRONUTRIENTS
Biotin

Nutritional supplements marketed to improve equine hoof quality virtually always include some quantity of biotin, and equine veterinarians and horse owners alike are widely aware of the link between this micronutrient and the health of the equine foot. Biotin is a water-soluble vitamin incorporated in its carboxylated form as a necessary cofactor into numerous enzymes involved in controlling diverse pathways of intermediary metabolism (such as gluconeogenesis, fatty acid synthesis, nucleic acid synthesis, and the urea cycle, to name a few), as well as cell proliferation and tissue growth. The daily biotin requirement for adult horses is met both through ingestion of this vitamin within the diet and, more importantly, through synthesis within the caudal gastrointestinal tract by the resident microbiota (this mechanism is likely responsible for the majority of biotin absorbed from the gastrointestinal tract and, in fact, there is no evidence that daily biotin requirements exceed the amount produced by these microbes in health).[67] As mentioned elsewhere in this article, biotin is routinely included in dietary supplements meant to improve hoof quality in horses, most often recommended for those individuals with brittle, damaged hoof horn; however, biotin deficiency *per se* is rarely established as the primary cause of poor hoof quality in this species.[68]

The therapeutic rationale for biotin supplementation to support improved hoof quality includes several mechanisms, including enhanced expression of cytokeratins associated with maturation and terminal differentiation of keratinocytes.[69] Supplementation has been evaluated in horses, and some of the therapeutic rationale for equine use has been supported by evidence from other species.[70–72] In general, treatment outcomes of these studies involve metrics of hoof growth rate and/or hoof quality/composition. One equine study demonstrated a significantly increased rate of hoof growth in ponies supplemented with biotin (0.12 mg/kg PO daily) for 5 months compared with unsupplemented ponies; in this study, older horses showed significantly lower growth rates than younger individuals as well.[58] Another study showed positive effects on hoof growth rate and hardness after 10 months of biotin supplementation, with some evidence of a dose–response effect.[73] A clinical trial evaluating the effect of biotin supplementation (20 mg/d for 9–38 months) on parameters associated with hoof horn quality (including hoof horn histology and tensile strength of horn at the bearing surface) suggested that horses receiving supplementation had improved hoof horn quality, both compared with their own pretreatment values, as well as to those of placebo-treated controls.[74] Further work from this same group demonstrated that oral biotin supplementation resulted in increased plasma biotin concentrations compared with placebo-treated controls; however, no difference in the hoof growth rate was observed.[75] Similar results were reported in another study of long-term oral biotin supplementation of 97 horses (5 mg/100–150 kg/d; 1–6 years), insofar as the metrics of hoof quality and tensile strength were improved but no effect on growth rate was noted.[76] Interestingly, in this particular study, hoof quality tangibly deteriorated in 7 of 10 horses after reduction or cessation of biotin administration, suggesting that this supplementation should likely be continuous in horses with abnormal hoof quality.[76] Although the results of these studies have varied, a consistent finding is the requirement for several months (at least) of supplementation before any treatment effect is observed.

Although strong evidence to support biotin supplementation to correct an established deficiency in horses is generally lacking, there does not seem to be a great deal of harm incurred in association with empiric supplementation and, indeed, this may be helpful for horses that have poor quality hoof horn in general. Being a water-soluble vitamin, large excesses of biotin are excreted in the urine and have not been associated with any reported clinical toxicity; doses of up to 30 mg/d are reportedly well-tolerated by mature horses.[68] For the purpose of improving hoof quality, supplementation with 0.03 to 0.04 mg/kg/d (which is 15–20 mg daily for a 500 kg horse) is reasonable, based on prevailing evidence.[68]

Selenium

Chronic selenium intoxication, or alkali disease, is one of the few nutritional excesses whose clinical signs are primarily displayed in keratinized structures (hair and hooves). This condition is associated with long-term, moderate (5–40 ppm) intake of selenium, generally at levels lower than those required to induce more severe, acute manifestations of selenium intoxication (acute death, blindness, ataxia, respiratory distress).[77] Horses are quite susceptible to chronic selenosis if exposed to selenium-rich forages for a prolonged period; in the United States, this is most likely to occur on the rangelands of Montana, Wyoming, Colorado, Utah, and North and South Dakota, where selenium-accumulating plants (such as *Astragalus, Stanleya, Oonopsis,* and *Xylorhiza* spp.) are relatively abundant, along with cyclic drought and alkaline soil.[78] Dried grass and alfalfa forages have also been implicated in chronic selenium intoxication events, occasionally in regions that are more typically considered marginally selenium deficient.[79] Areas such as the Pacific Northwest and Great Lakes regions of the United States are generally selenium-deficient, making the toxicity that occurs in these areas more likely to be related to iatrogenic causes, including overzealous supplementation.

The daily dietary selenium requirement for adult horses can be met by feeding a ration containing 0.1 to 0.2 ppm selenium (corresponding with approximately 1 mg elemental selenium per horse per day), with little rationale for supplementation in excess of 0.5 ppm.[68] Dietary selenium levels of as low as 5 ppm (5 mg/kg dry matter) can cause induction of clinical alkali disease, the signs of which include loss of mane/tail hairs, cracking of the hoof wall near the coronary band, and, in more severe cases, sloughing of the hoof capsules. An upper safe limit of dietary selenium content of 5 ppm has been recommended, but 2 ppm is likely more advisable (and still well in excess of NRC recommendations).[68]

The lesions of chronic selenosis are suggestive, particularly if multiple horses in a particular cohort are similarly affected. Confirmation of the diagnosis historically has been performed by measuring serum, plasma, or whole blood selenium concentrations or whole blood glutathione peroxidase activity in affected horses. The measurement of the hepatic selenium concentration is useful for biopsy or postmortem confirmation of chronic exposure. Additionally, recent work suggests that equine hair samples can be analyzed and used to evaluate an individual's selenium exposure for up to 3 years after initial exposure to high-risk feedstuffs; this technique may be a useful minimally invasive technique for the investigation of chronic herd problems.[80]

Copper and Zinc

Zinc is directly involved in skin, hair, and hoof development (among many other functions throughout the body), and dietary zinc deficiency is associated with hair loss, parakeratotic hyperkeratosis of the skin (particularly of the lower limbs), and abnormal collagen production. A dietary zinc requirement of 40 mg/kg dry matter seems to be adequate for adult horses, and horses seem to be fairly tolerant of large amounts of zinc in the diet (although this excess is not recommended, dietary zinc levels of 500–700 mg/kg feed have been reportedly well-tolerated).[68] Perhaps a more pressing concern related to a high levels of dietary zinc is the associated potential to interfere with dietary copper absorption.[81] Copper is a cofactor for several enzymes involved in the metabolism of collagen and other extracellular matrix components, as well as antioxidant capacity, melanin synthesis, and many other functions. Copper deficiency has a clearly demonstrated association with developmental orthopedic disease in horses, forming the basis of recommendations to carefully attend to copper concentrations in broodmare diets. A level of 10 mg Cu/kg dry matter seems to be appropriate for adult horses; as with zinc, horses seem to be very tolerant of large amounts of copper in the diet (again, although not recommended, >700 mg Cu/kg dry matter has been fed to pregnant pony mares with no significant adverse effects noted in the mares or their foals[82]). Zinc deficiency is associated with poor hoof quality in horses and is perhaps more likely to be observed in young animals, but neither copper nor zinc have received significant investigation for their roles in promoting hoof health in this species. That said, an assessment of dietary zinc and copper levels (as well as the composition of the diet in general) should likely be performed in horses with poor hoof quality before attempting empiric supplementation of specific micronutrients.

ROLE OF BODY CONDITION

Although not directly related to composition of the diet, another nutritional influence on the foot that is increasingly well-established is that of persistent caloric excess that results in obesity. Nutritional obesity is well-known to be associated with (potentially) reversible tissue insulin resistance,[83–85] and excess body mass can influence the magnitude of structural injury incurred during a bout of laminitis owing to any cause[86]; the relevance of both of these changes has been clarified through the work of several research groups over the last 15 years (some of which is discussed elsewhere in this review). However, a relatively unexplored mechanism by which white adipose tissue can directly affect the health of the foot is through its own activity as an endocrine organ. Elaboration of adipokines, such as leptin and adiponectin, is well-known to influence satiety, insulin sensitivity, and metabolism, among other things, in multiple species (including horses) and has been shown to consistently vary in proportion to adiposity.[87–89] More recently, investigation of leptin's role in certain dermatologic conditions associated with obesity and insulin resistance in humans (such as skin tag and acanthosis nigricans) has revealed the degree to which keratinocyte biology can be influenced by leptin, both that delivered to the tissue in an endocrine fashion and that produced locally by keratinocytes themselves.[90,91]

Although difficult to extract from its many connections to insulin and insulin resistance, leptin may also act synergistically with, or even independent of, insulin to drive pathophysiology within the equine digital lamellae. Observational studies of pony populations that originally identified hyperinsulinemia as a strongly predictive risk factor for laminitis also at the same time identified hyperleptinemia as being linked to that risk,[9] and obese equids with ID are typically concurrently hyperleptinemic.[49,92,93] Equine digital lamellar keratinocytes express leptin receptor, and leptin can be acutely regulated by factors other than adiposity in humans and horses (eg, leptin concentrations increase acutely during a euglycemic–hyperinsulinemic clamp procedure).[94–98] Leptin can influence the proinflammatory response of keratinocytes and promote epithelial-to-mesenchymal transition, both of which have been implicated in the pathogenesis of equine laminitis.[99–102] Moreover, elaboration of leptin locally by epithelial cells themselves[103,104] can be induced by tension or stretch in vitro[105]; a local paracrine effect in response to mechanical changes within the tissue is plausible and seems particularly relevant in the setting of laminitis, given the mechanical forces to which lamellar keratinocytes are exposed. Given the effects that leptin has on epithelial cells in other species and systems, as well as what is known regarding the regulation of leptin in obese equids with ID, a more critical evaluation of the role of leptin and other adipokines in the pathophysiology of equine laminitis is needed. In the meantime, as mentioned elsewhere in this article, weight loss should be encouraged in overweight or obese horses in an expedient manner to improve insulin and glucose dynamics and minimize risk of laminitis.

DISCLOSURE

The author has nothing to disclose.

REFERENCES

1. van Eps AW, Burns TA. Are there shared mechanisms in the pathophysiology of different clinical forms of laminitis and what are the implications for prevention and treatment? Vet Clin North Am Equine Pract 2019;35(2):379–98.

2. Argo CM. Nutritional management of the older horse. Vet Clin North Am Equine Pract 2016;32(2):343–54.

3. Burden FA, Bell N. Donkey nutrition and malnutrition. Vet Clin North Am Equine Pract 2019;35(3):469–79.

4. Geor RJ. Pasture-associated laminitis. Vet Clin North Am Equine Pract 2009; 25(1):39–50, v–vi.

5. Harris P, Bailey SR, Elliott J, et al. Countermeasures for pasture-associated laminitis in ponies and horses. J Nutr 2006;136(7 Suppl):2114S–21S.

6. Harris P, Geor RJ. Primer on dietary carbohydrates and utility of the glycemic index in equine nutrition. Vet Clin North Am Equine Pract 2009;25(1):23–37, v.

7. Harris PA, Ellis AD, Fradinho MJ, et al. Review: feeding conserved forage to horses: recent advances and recommendations. Animal 2017;11(6):958–67.

8. Ralston SL. Evidence-based equine nutrition. Vet Clin North Am Equine Pract 2007;23(2):365–84.

9. Carter RA, Treiber KH, Geor RJ, et al. Prediction of incipient pasture-associated laminitis from hyperinsulinaemia, hyperleptinaemia and generalised and localised obesity in a cohort of ponies. Equine Vet J 2009;41(2):171–8.

10. Treiber KH, Kronfeld DS, Geor RJ. Insulin resistance in equids: possible role in laminitis. J Nutr 2006;136(7 Suppl):2094S–8S.

11. Treiber KH, Kronfeld DS, Hess TM, et al. Evaluation of genetic and metabolic predispositions and nutritional risk factors for pasture-associated laminitis in ponies. J Am Vet Med Assoc 2006;228(10):1538–45.

12. Asplin KE, Sillence MN, Pollitt CC, et al. Induction of laminitis by prolonged hyperinsulinaemia in clinically normal ponies. Vet J 2007;174(3):530–5.

13. de Laat MA, McGowan CM, Sillence MN, et al. Equine laminitis: induced by 48 h hyperinsulinaemia in standardbred horses. Equine Vet J 2010;42(2):129–35.

14. De Meyts P. The insulin receptor and its signal transduction network. In: Feingold KR, Anawalt B, Boyce A, et al, editors. Endotext. South Dartmouth (MA): MDText.com, Inc; 2000. NBK378978 [bookaccession].

15. de Laat MA, Sillence MN, McGowan CM, et al. Continuous intravenous infusion of glucose induces endogenous hyperinsulinaemia and lamellar histopathology in standardbred horses. Vet J 2012;191(3):317–22.

16. de Laat MA, Patterson-Kane JC, Pollitt CC, et al. Histological and morphometric lesions in the pre-clinical, developmental phase of insulin-induced laminitis in standardbred horses. Vet J 2013;195(3):305–12.

17. Stokes SM, Belknap JK, Engiles JB, et al. Continuous digital hypothermia prevents lamellar failure in the euglycaemic hyperinsulinemic clamp model of equine laminitis. Equine Vet J 2019;51(5):658–4.

18. Burns TA, Watts MR, Weber PS, et al. Distribution of insulin receptor and insulin-like growth factor-1 receptor in the digital laminae of mixed-breed ponies: an immunohistochemical study. Equine Vet J 2013;45(3):326–32.

19. de Laat MA, Pollitt CC, Kyaw-Tanner MT, et al. A potential role for lamellar insulin-like growth factor-1 receptor in the pathogenesis of hyperinsulinaemic laminitis. Vet J 2013;197(2):302–6.

20. Rahnama S, Vathsangam N, Spence R, et al. Identification of monoclonal antibodies suitable for blocking IGF-1 receptors in the horse. Domest Anim Endocrinol 2021;74:106510.

21. Rahnama S, Spence R, Vathsangam N, et al. Effects of insulin on IGF-1 receptors in equine lamellar tissue in vitro. Domest Anim Endocrinol 2021;74:106530.

22. Rahnama S, Vathsangam N, Spence R, et al. Effects of an anti-IGF-1 receptor monoclonal antibody on laminitis induced by prolonged hyperinsulinaemia in standardbred horses. PLoS One 2020;15:e0239261.

23. Wattle O, Pollitt CC. Lamellar metabolism. Clin Tech Eq Pract 2004;3:22–33.

24. Asplin KE, Curlewis JD, McGowan CM, et al. Glucose transport in the equine hoof. Equine Vet J 2011;43(2):196–201.

25. de laat MA, Clement CK, Sillence MN, et al. The impact of prolonged hyperinsulinemia on glucose transport in equine skeletal muscle and digital lamellae. Equine Vet J 2015;47(4):494–501.

26. Pinnell EF, Belknap JK, Burns TA, et al. Glucose attenuates AMPK signaling in the absence of insulin in equine digital lamellae. J Vet Intern Med 2020;34(6): 2830–989.

27. Wang L, Pawlak EA, Johnson PJ, et al. Impact of laminitis on the canonical wnt signaling pathway in basal epithelial cells of the equine digital laminae. PLoS One 2013;8(2):e56025 (TRUNCATED).

28. Aroeira LS, Loureiro J, González-Mateo GT, et al. Characterization of epithelial-to-mesenchymal transition of mesothelial cells in a mouse model of chronic peritoneal exposure to high glucose dialysate. Perit Dial Int 2008;28(Suppl 5): S29–33.

29. Lv ZM, Wang Q, Wan Q, et al. The role of the p38 MAPK signaling pathway in high glucose-induced epithelial-mesenchymal transition of cultured human renal tubular epithelial cells. PLoS One 2011;6(7):e22806.

30. Lee YJ, Han HJ. Troglitazone ameliorates high glucose-induced EMT and dysfunction of SGLTs through PI3K/akt, GSK-3β, Snail1, and β-catenin in renal proximal tubule cells. Am J Physiol Ren Physiol 2010;298(5):F1263–75.

31. Hoffman RM. Carbohydrates. In: Geor RJ, Harris PA, Coenen M, editors. Equine applied and clinical nutrition: health, welfare, and performance.. 1st edition. St. Louis: Saunders; 2013. p. 156–67.

32. Borgia L, Valberg S, McCue M, et al. Glycaemic and insulinaemic responses to feeding hay with different non-structural carbohydrate content in control and polysaccharide storage myopathy-affected horses. J Anim Physiol Anim Nutr (Berl) 2011;95(6):798–807.

33. Zeyner A, Hoffmeister C, Einspanier A, et al. Glycaemic and insulinaemic response of quarter horses to concentrates high in fat and low in soluble carbohydrates. Equine Vet J Suppl 2006;(36):643–7.

34. Hoffman RM, Boston RC, Stefanovski D, et al. Obesity and diet affect glucose dynamics and insulin sensitivity in thoroughbred geldings. J Anim Sci 2003; 81(9):2333–42.

35. Rapson JL, Schott HC 2nd, Nielsen BD, et al. Effects of age and diet on glucose and insulin dynamics in the horse. Equine Vet J 2018;50(5):690–6.

36. Moore-Colyer MJ, Lumbis K, Longland A, et al. The effect of five different wetting treatments on the nutrient content and microbial concentration in hay for horses. PLoS One 2014;9(11):e114079.

37. Carslake HB, Argo CM, Pinchbeck GL, et al. Insulinaemic and glycaemic responses to three forages in ponies. Vet J 2018;235:83–9.

38. Argo CM, Dugdale AH, McGowan CM. Considerations for the use of restricted, soaked grass hay diets to promote weight loss in the management of equine metabolic syndrome and obesity. Vet J 2015;206(2):170–7.

39. Moore-Colyer M, Longland A, Harris P, et al. Mapping the bacterial ecology on the phyllosphere of dry and post soaked grass hay for horses. PLoS One 2020; 15(1):e0227151.

40. Longland AC, Barfoot C, Harris PA. Effect of period, water temperature and agitation on loss of water-soluble carbohydrates and protein from grass hay: implications for equine feeding management. Vet Rec 2014;174(3):68.

41. Longland AC, Barfoot C, Harris PA. Effects of soaking on the water-soluble carbohydrate and crude protein content of hay. Vet.Rec. 2011;168(23):618.

42. Owens TG, Barnes M, Gargano VM, et al. Nutrient content changes from steaming or soaking timothy-alfalfa hay: effects on feed preferences and acute glycemic response in standardbred racehorses1. J Anim Sci 2019;97(10):4199–207.

43. Longland AC, Byrd BM. Pasture nonstructural carbohydrates and equine laminitis. J Nutr 2006;136(7 Suppl):2099S–102S.

44. Longland AC, Barfoot C, Harris PA. Effects of grazing muzzles on intakes of dry matter and water-soluble carbohydrates by ponies grazing spring, summer, and autumn swards, as well as autumn swards of different heights. J Equine Vet Sci 2016;40:26–33.

45. de Laat MA, Hampson BA, Sillence MN, et al. Sustained, low-intensity exercise achieved by a dynamic feeding system decreases body fat in ponies. J Vet Intern Med 2016;30(5):1732–8.

46. Bamford NJ, Potter SJ, Baskerville CL, et al. Influence of dietary restriction and low-intensity exercise on weight loss and insulin sensitivity in obese equids. J Vet Intern Med 2019;33(1).

47. Glunk EC, Hathaway MR, Grev AM, et al. The effect of a limit-fed diet and slow-feed hay nets on morphometric measurements and postprandial metabolite and hormone patterns in adult horses. J Anim Sci 2015;93(8):4144–52.

48. Longland AC, Barfoot C, Harris PA. Strip-grazing: reduces pony dry matter intakes and changes in bodyweight and morphometrics. Equine Vet J 2020.

49. Durham AE, Frank N, McGowan CM, et al. ECEIM consensus statement on equine metabolic syndrome. J Vet Intern Med 2019;33(2):335–49.

50. Geor RJ, Harris P. Dietary management of obesity and insulin resistance: countering risk for laminitis. Vet Clin North Am Equine Pract 2009;25(1):51–65, vi.

51. Freestone JF, Wolfsheimer KJ, Ford RB, et al. Triglyceride, insulin, and cortisol responses of ponies to fasting and dexamethasone administration. J Vet Intern Med 1991;5(1):15–22.

52. Frank N, Sojka JE, Latour MA. Effect of withholding feed on concentration and composition of plasma very low density lipoprotein and serum nonesterified fatty acids in horses. Am J Vet Res 2002;63(7):1018–21.

53. Dunkel B, Wilford SA, Parkinson NJ, et al. Severe hypertriglyceridaemia in horses and ponies with endocrine disorders. Equine Vet J 2014;46(1):118–22.

54. Crandell KG, Pagan JD, Harris P, et al. A comparison of grain, oil and beet pulp as energy sources for the exercised horse. Equine Vet J Suppl 1999;30:485–9.

55. Lindberg JE, Karlsson CP. Effect of partial replacement of oats with sugar beet pulp and maize oil on nutrient utilisation in horses. Equine Vet J 2001;33(6): 585–90.

56. Williams CA, Kronfeld DS, Staniar WB, et al. Plasma glucose and insulin responses of thoroughbred mares fed a meal high in starch and sugar or fat and fiber. J Anim Sci 2001;79(8):2196–201.

57. Hoffman RM, Kronfeld DS, Cooper WL, et al. Glucose clearance in grazing mares is affected by diet, pregnancy, and lactation. J Anim Sci 2003;81(7): 1764–71.

58. Reilly JD, Hopegood L, Gould L, et al. Effect of a supplementary dietary evening primrose oil mixture on hoof growth, hoof growth rate and hoof lipid fractions in horses: a controlled and blinded trial. Equine Vet J Suppl 1998;26:58–65.

59. Valberg SJ. Muscle conditions affecting sport horses. Vet Clin North Am Equine Pract 2018;34(2):253–76.

60. Ekfalck A, Appelgren LE, Funkquist B, et al. Distribution of labelled cysteine and methionine in the matrix of the stratum medium of the wall and in the laminar layer of the equine hoof. Zentralbl Veterinarmed A 1990;37(7):481–91.

61. Mok CH, Urschel KL. Amino acid requirements in horses. Asian-Australas J Anim Sci 2020;33(5):679–95.

62. Sticker LS, Thompson DL, Gentry LR. Pituitary hormone and insulin responses to infusion of amino acids and N-methyl-D,L-aspartate in horses. J Anim Sci 2001;79(3):735–44.

63. Fowden AL, Comline RS, Silver M. Insulin secretion and carbohydrate metabolism during pregnancy in the mare. Equine Vet J 1984;16(4):239–46.

64. Fowden AL, Gardner DS, Ousey JC, et al. Maturation of pancreatic beta-cell function in the fetal horse during late gestation. J Endocrinol 2005;186(3): 467–73.

65. Loos CMM, Dorsch SC, Elzinga SE, et al. A high protein meal affects plasma insulin concentrations and amino acid metabolism in horses with equine metabolic syndrome. Vet J 2019;251:105341.

66. Manfredi JM, Stapley ED, Nadeau JA, et al. Investigation of the effects of a dietary supplement on insulin and adipokine concentrations in equine metabolic syndrome/insulin dysregulation. J Equine Vet Sci 2020;88:102930.

67. Zeyner A, Harris P. Ch. 9: vitamins. In: Geor R, Harris P, Coenen M, editors. Equine applied and clinical nutrition: health, welfare, and performance. 1st edition. St. Louis, MO: Saunders; 2013. p. 183–4.

68. NRC (National Research Council). In: Lawrence LM, Cymbaluk NF, Freeman DW, et al, editors. Nutrient requirements of horses. 6th edition. Washington, DC: The National Academies Press; 2007.

69. Fritsche A, Mathis GA, Althaus FR. Pharmacologic effects of biotin on epidermal cells. Schweiz Arch Tierheilkd 1991;133(6):277–83.

70. Colombo VE, Gerber F, Bronhofer M, et al. Treatment of brittle fingernails and onychoschizia with biotin: scanning electron microscopy. J Am Acad Dermatol 1990;23(6 Pt 1):1127–32.

71. Comben N, Clark RJ, Sutherland DJ. Clinical observations on the response of equine hoof defects to dietary supplementation with biotin. Vet Rec 1984; 115(25–26):642–5.

72. Webb NG, Penny RH, Johnston AM. Effect of a dietary supplement of biotin on pig hoof horn strength and hardness. Vet Rec 1984;114(8):185–9.

73. Buffa EA, Van Den Berg SS, Verstraete FJ, et al. Effect of dietary biotin supplement on equine hoof horn growth rate and hardness. Equine Vet J 1992;24(6): 472–4.

74. Zenker W, Josseck H, Geyer H. Histological and physical assessment of poor hoof horn quality in Lipizzaner horses and a therapeutic trial with biotin and a placebo. Equine Vet J 1995;27(3):183–91.

75. Josseck H, Zenker W, Geyer H. Hoof horn abnormalities in Lipizzaner horses and the effect of dietary biotin on macroscopic aspects of hoof horn quality. Equine Vet J 1995;27(3):175–82.

76. Geyer H, Schulze J. The long-term influence of biotin supplementation on hoof horn quality in horses. Schweiz Arch Tierheilkd 1994;136(4):137–49.

77. Mihajlović M. Selenium toxicity in domestic animals. Glas Srp Akad Nauka Med 1992;(42):131–44.

78. Anonymous U. Selenium-accumulating plants. Available at: https://www.ars. usda.gov/pacific-west-area/logan-ut/poisonous-plant-research/docs/selenium-accumulating-plants/#:~:text=Plants%20that%20will%20accumulate%20selenium,barley%2C%20wheat%2C%20and%20alfalfa. Accessed February 8, 2021.

79. Witte ST, Will LA, Olsen CR, et al. Chronic selenosis in horses fed locally produced alfalfa hay. J Am Vet Med Assoc 1993;202(3):406–9.

80. Davis TZ, Stegelmeier BL, Hall JO. Analysis in horse hair as a means of evaluating selenium toxicoses and long-term exposures. J Agric Food Chem 2014; 62(30):7393–7.

81. Bridges CH, Moffitt PG. Influence of variable content of dietary zinc on copper metabolism of weanling foals. Am J Vet Res 1990;51(2):275–80.

82. Smith JD, Jordan RM, Nelson ML. Tolerance of ponies to high levels of dietary copper. J Anim Sci 1975;41(6):1645–9.

83. Carter RA, McCutcheon LJ, George LA, et al. Effects of diet-induced weight gain on insulin sensitivity and plasma hormone and lipid concentrations in horses. Am J Vet Res 2009;70(10):1250–8.

84. Carter R, McCutcheon LJ, Burns TA, et al. Increased adiposity in horses is associated with decreased insulin sensitivity but unchanged inflammatory cytokine expression in subcutaneous adipose tissue. Proc Forum Am Coll Vet Intern Med 2008;22(3):735.

85. Bamford NJ, Potter SJ, Harris PA, et al. Effect of increased adiposity on insulin sensitivity and adipokine concentrations in horses and ponies fed a high fat diet, with or without a once daily high glycaemic meal. Equine Vet J 2016;48(3): 368–73.

86. Leise BS, Faleiros RR, Watts M, et al. Hindlimb laminar inflammatory response is similar to that present in forelimbs after carbohydrate overload in horses. Equine Vet J 2012;44(6):633–9.

87. Schultz N, Geor RJ, Manfredi JM. Factors associated with leptin and adiponectin concentrations in a large across breed cohort of horses and ponies. J Vet Intern Med 2014;28:998.

88. Kearns CF, McKeever KH, Roegner V, et al. Adiponectin and leptin are related to fat mass in horses. Vet J 2006;172(3):460–5.

89. Buff PR, Dodds AC, Morrison CD, et al. Leptin in horses: tissue localization and relationship between peripheral concentrations of leptin and body condition. J Anim Sci 2002;80(11):2942–8.

90. Seleit I, Bakry OA, Samaka RM, et al. Immunohistochemical evaluation of leptin role in skin tags. Ultrastruct Pathol 2015;39(4):235–44.

91. Atwa M, Emara A, Balata M, et al. Serum leptin, adiponectin, and resistin among adult patients with acanthosis nigricans: correlations with insulin resistance and risk factors for cardiovascular disease. Int J Dermatol 2014;53(10):e410–20.

92. Frank N. Equine metabolic syndrome. Vet Clin North Am Equine Pract 2011; 27(1):73–92.

93. Frank N, Elliott SB, Brandt LE, et al. Physical characteristics, blood hormone concentrations, and plasma lipid concentrations in obese horses with insulin resistance. J Am Vet Med Assoc 2006;228(9):1383–90.

94. Nijveldt E, Watts MR, Belknap JK, et al. Systemic and local regulation of leptin in a model of endocrinopathic laminitis. J Vet Intern Med 2019;33(5):2375–547.

95. Faraj M, Beauregard G, Tardif A, et al. Regulation of leptin, adiponectin and acylation-stimulating protein by hyperinsulinaemia and hyperglycaemia in vivo in healthy lean young men. Diabetes Metab 2008;34(4 Pt 1):334–42.

96. Pratley RE, Nicolson M, Bogardus C, et al. Effects of acute hyperinsulinemia on plasma leptin concentrations in insulin-sensitive and insulin-resistant pima indians. J Clin Endocrinol Metab 1996;81(12):4418–21.

97. Pratley RE, Ren K, Milner MR, et al. Insulin increases leptin mRNA expression in abdominal subcutaneous adipose tissue in humans. Mol Genet Metab 2000; 70(1):19–26.

98. Malmström R, Taskinen MR, Karonen SL, et al. Insulin increases plasma leptin concentrations in normal subjects and patients with NIDDM. Diabetologia 1996;39(8):993–6.

99. Lee M, Lee E, Jin SH, et al. Leptin regulates the pro-inflammatory response in human epidermal keratinocytes. Arch Dermatol Res 2018;310(4):351–62.

100. Watts MR, Hegedus OC, Eades SC, et al. Association of sustained supraphysiologic hyperinsulinemia and inflammatory signaling within the digital lamellae in light-breed horses. J Vet Intern Med 2019;33(3):1483–92.

101. Leise BS, Watts M, Tanhoff E, et al. Laminar regulation of STAT1 and STAT3 in black walnut extract and carbohydrate overload induced models of laminitis. J Vet Intern Med 2012;26(4):996–1004.

102. Dern K, Burns TA, Watts MR, et al. Influence of digital hypothermia on lamellar events related to IL-6/gp130 signalling in equine sepsis-related laminitis. Equine Vet J 2020;52(3):441–8.

103. Iguchi M, Aiba S, Yoshino Y, et al. Human follicular papilla cells carry out non-adipose tissue production of leptin. J Invest Dermatol 2001;117(6):1349–56.

104. Murad A, Nath AK, Cha ST, et al. Leptin is an autocrine/paracrine regulator of wound healing. FASEB J 2003;17(13):1895–7.

105. Chiu CZ, Wang BW, Shyu KG. Angiotensin II and the ERK pathway mediate the induction of leptin by mechanical cyclic stretch in cultured rat neonatal cardiomyocytes. Clin Sci (Lond) 2014;126(7):483–95.

Cryotherapy Techniques
Best Protocols to Support the Foot in Health and Disease

Daniela Luethy, DVM

KEYWORDS

- Laminitis • Ice • Cryotherapy • Digit • Hoof • Hypothermia

KEY POINTS

- Distal limb hypothermia induces vasoconstriction, analgesia, anti-inflammatory effects, and hypometabolism within tissues.
- Distal limb cryotherapy is currently one of the best therapeutic interventions available to veterinarians to help prevent the development of laminitis and to help treat acute laminitis in the early stages, with studies showing that cryotherapy reduces the severity of sepsis-related laminitis and hyperinsulinemic laminitis in experimental models and reduces the incidence of laminitis in clinical colitis cases.
- Current literature supports the use of immersion of the entire hoof and a portion of the distal limb in ice and water, a sleeve-style ice boot that does not incorporate the foot, and a prototype dry sleeve boot for application of distal limb cryotherapy in horses.

DEFINITIONS

- Cryotherapy: cold therapy, the local or general application of cold temperatures
- Hypothermia: abnormally low temperature

INTRODUCTION

Laminitis is a devastating disease, which accounts for significant morbidity and mortality in horses.[1] Laminitis can occur owing to sepsis-related conditions, as well as to endocrinopathies, such as equine metabolic syndrome and pituitary pars intermedia dysfunction. Treatment of equine laminitis continues to be a challenge despite recent advancements in the understanding of the pathophysiology of laminitis. Since the previous *Veterinary Clinics of North America: Equine Practice* article discussing equine digital cryotherapy published a decade ago, significant advances have been achieved, expanding the knowledge of the use of digital cryotherapy in laminitis.[1] With more

Large Animal Medicine, Department of Large Animal Clinical Sciences, University of Florida, College of Veterinary Medicine, PO Box 100136, Gainesville, FL 32610-0136, USA
E-mail address: dluethy@ufl.edu

Vet Clin Equine 37 (2021) 685–693
https://doi.org/10.1016/j.cveq.2021.07.005
0749-0739/21/© 2021 Elsevier Inc. All rights reserved.

evidence supporting its use, distal limb hypothermia or cryotherapy has become a standard of care for both prevention of laminitis and treatment of the acute phases of laminitis.[1,2]

BACKGROUND

Cryotherapy originated thousands of years ago. Ancient Egyptians recognized the anti-inflammatory and analgesic effects of cryotherapy.[3] Cryotherapy has been commonly used in veterinary medicine for conditions such as soft tissue injuries in humans and performance injuries in horses,[4,5] and more recently for laminitis in horses.

Effects of Hypothermia on Tissues

Hypothermia's effects on tissues remain incompletely understood. Hypothermia produces analgesic and anti-inflammatory effects. Furthermore, it induces alterations in vascular tone and a reduced metabolic rate in tissues.[4] Hypothermia stimulates profound local vasoconstriction, most significantly through sympathetic nervous control as well as a direct constriction of vessel walls.[4] Cryotherapy applied to the equine digit has been shown to decrease soft tissue perfusion.[6] Interestingly, in other species, a reflex intermittent vasodilation, referred to as a "hunting reaction," occurs associated with cryotherapy; however, this has not been documented in horses.[6,7] This reaction is attributed to dilation of blood vessels in muscular tissue, and it is possible that the lack of skeletal muscle tissue in the distal limb of horses may explain the lack of this "hunting reaction" response to cryotherapy.[6,7] In addition, a vast vascular network within the hoof can create rapid net perfusion changes. Cryotherapy applied to the equine distal limb produces profound vasoconstriction within the digit, with a scintigraphic study demonstrating a significant reduction in perfusion after 30 minutes of ice water immersion.[6] Hypothermia also acts directly on peripheral nerves to prolong the refractory period, slow conduction velocity, and increase stimulation threshold, thereby decreasing sensitivity of the tissues.[8]

In addition, hypothermia induces anti-inflammatory effects by reducing the production and activity of proinflammatory cytokines, increasing the production of anti-inflammatory cytokines, and reducing the production of oxygen free radicals.[9–11] In rats, hypothermia has been shown to produce anti-inflammatory effects in sepsis and systemic inflammatory response syndrome (SIRS) models.[10,12]

In addition, hypothermia inhibits the metabolism of tissues, with studies showing a direct relationship between temperature and tissue metabolic rate and oxygen consumption.[13] Hypothermia has been shown to have neuroprotective effects after ischemic or traumatic brain injury, with a reduction in oxygen, glucose, and metabolites required by the hypothermic tissue, inducing enhanced survival of the tissue during ischemic periods.[14]

Potential Adverse Effects of Hypothermia

No intervention is without the potential for adverse effects. Hypothermia may be associated with coagulopathy and increased infection risk, whereas whole body hypothermia can result in derangement of cardiac, metabolic, or endocrine function.[15] In humans, local hypothermia adverse effects are rare, consisting of frostbite or nerve palsy.[16] In addition, placement of the distal limb in a cool, moist environment for a prolonged period of time can induce immersion foot or trench foot in humans.[17] In contrast to humans, the equine distal limb is tolerant of prolonged periods of hypothermia with minimal adverse consequences, providing an excellent opportunity for the use of cryotherapy. The equine distal limb lacks significant musculature and contains superficial major blood vessels, producing an ideal state for induction of hypothermia in the foot, but the horses' hair coat and hoof create a barrier for effective heat conduction and exchange. Further discussion of the potential adverse effects of cryotherapy in horses is found later.

Proposed Mechanisms of the Benefits of Hypothermia in Equine Laminitis

Although the exact pathophysiology of laminitis remains incompletely understood and is likely multifactorial, research supports an association between hyperinsulinemia and endocrinopathic laminitis.[18] The effects of hypothermia on tissue discussed above represent potential mechanisms for the beneficial effects of cryotherapy noted in equine laminitis.[1,19] Cryotherapy induces profound vasoconstriction, which may limit the delivery of laminitis trigger factors to the foot via circulation. Cryotherapy decreases tissue metabolic rate, which may reduce the production and activation of lamellar matrix metalloproteinases (MMPs) and inhibit enzymatic degradation of lamellae by these MMPs. Furthermore, this hypometabolism may protect lamellae from ischemic injury and reduce local proinflammatory cytokine production and activity. Inflammatory injury within the lamellae may be caused by penetration of polymorphonuclear leukocytes (PMNs), and the vasoconstriction and decreased metabolic rate produced by cryotherapy may reduce PMN activity.

SUPPORT FOR THE USE OF DISTAL LIMB CRYOTHERAPY IN EQUINE LAMINITIS

Based on human recommendations, the initial duration of cryotherapy in horses was similar to human medicine, generally limited to 30 to 45 minutes.[19] These recommendations were based on an attempt to avoid frostbite and nerve palsy, although these adverse effects were not noted in horses with their feet immersed in snow in winter conditions.[7] Pollitt and Eps evaluated continuous, prolonged (48 hours) distal limb cryotherapy in 4 adult Standardbred horses using a slurry of crushed ice and water and a boot encompassing the entire hoof and distal limb.[7] They found that this continuous cryotherapy was well tolerated, resulting in no adverse effects in the horses studied, despite direct skin contact with an ice water slurry. Application of the ice boot rapidly decreased the hoof temperature and achieved mean temperatures of less than 5°C for the duration of application. Following this work, continuous application of cryotherapy began to be used more commonly in equine practice.

The efficacy of digital cryotherapy was first evaluated in a grain overload model in 6 Standardbred horses.[19] Cryotherapy was well tolerated and effective in cooling the feet, and laminitis histology scores were significantly less in the treated limb than the contralateral untreated limb. In addition, MMP-2 messenger RNA (mRNA) expression was lower in the treated feet than the untreated feet. The investigators postulated that the primary mechanism of action was vasoconstriction and hypometabolism induced by the cryotherapy preventing delivery of hematogenous laminitis trigger factors and reducing lamellar MMP activity.[19] Building on this work, the investigators conducted a study of 18 Standardbred horses in an oligofructose laminitis induction model. Seventy-two hours of distal limb cryotherapy resulted in reduced lameness and lower laminitis histology scores than in untreated controls, supporting the use of distal limb cryotherapy in the development phases of laminitis.[20]

Further research into the use of distal limb cryotherapy has supported its use after clinical signs of laminitis have already begun. One study evaluated application of distal limb cryotherapy after lameness was detected in an oligofructose model of laminitis in 8 Standardbred horses.[21] Once lameness was detected at a walk, continuous digital cryotherapy was applied to 1 limb, whereas the other limb was left untreated. Similar to previous research, histology scores were reduced in the treated limbs as compared with the untreated limbs, demonstrating reduction in the severity of lamellar injury by distal limb cryotherapy even when applied after the detection of lameness in an acute laminitis model. This study supported the use of cryotherapy as a treatment for acute laminitis even after lameness has developed.

Clinical applications have also supported the use of prophylactic digital cryotherapy. A multicenter retrospective case series evaluated the development of laminitis in 130 horses diagnosed with colitis.[22] Ten percent of horses who were treated with prophylactic digital cryotherapy developed laminitis, as compared with 33% of horses that did not receive cryotherapy, resulting in a 10 times lower odds of developing laminitis in the treated horses as compared with untreated horses.[22]

The mechanisms for reduction of laminitis in models of laminitis are not completely understood. One study found profound inhibition of inflammatory mediators when cryotherapy was initiated before sepsis or laminitis, suggesting that cryotherapy may limit lamellar injury through anti-inflammatory effects.[23] However, a subsequent study whereby cryotherapy was initiated at the time of clinical lameness did not show this inhibition of inflammatory mediators, while still having a protective effect on the lamellae.[24] In an oligofructose laminitis model of sepsis-related laminitis whereby distal limb cryotherapy was applied at the onset of clinical signs of sepsis, 2 inflammatory mediators (IL-6 and COX-2) and lamellar leukocyte numbers were decreased with cryotherapy, suggesting a more focused inhibition of inflammatory signaling when initiated at the clinical onset of sepsis.[25]

A significant proportion of the early literature evaluating cryotherapy for laminitis in horses used the oligofructose model for sepsis-related laminitis, and its applicability to endocrinopathic laminitis was not well understood. A more recent study evaluated the euglycemic hyperinsulinemic clamp (EHC) model of endocrinopathic laminitis.[26] Eight Standardbred horses underwent laminitis induction with the EHC model, with 1 limb treated with continuous digital cryotherapy before recognition of lameness and the contralateral limb untreated. The treated limbs had lower histology scores than the untreated limbs and did not display lesions compatible with lamellar failure seen in the untreated limbs, supporting the use of continuous cryotherapy to reduce the severity of laminitis in the EHC model, and therefore, potential for prevention and treatment of endocrinopathic laminitis.[26] Further research demonstrated decreased levels of lamellar mRNA levels in treated limbs compared with untreated limbs, further supporting the use of digital cryotherapy as a first-line treatment for acute laminitis associated with hyperinsulinemia in horses.[27]

Most studies evaluating digital cryotherapy in equine research models have not reported significant adverse effects. However, in a clinical population, the potential for adverse effects was noted anecdotally. To further evaluate this clinical finding, a 2018 multicenter retrospective study of sleeve-style digital cryotherapy was performed in 285 hospitalized horses and identified pathologic conditions secondary to this method of hypothermia in 7% of horses.[28] Furthermore, longer duration of cryotherapy was associated with an increased incidence of pathologic conditions, including dermatitis, cellulitis, alopecia, coronitis, tissue necrosis, and distal limb edema. Horses undergoing 0 to 36 hours of cryotherapy had an incidence of pathologic lesions of 13%, whereas horses undergoing cryotherapy for greater than 72 hours had an incidence of 39%. Lesions were purported to be similar to frostbite and prolonged water immersion injuries noted in other species. Therefore, recommendations now include close monitoring for dermal injury in horses where prolonged wet cryotherapy is used. In the author's hospital, they often implement a 1-to 2-hour period every 24 hours whereby the ice boots are removed, and the limbs are thoroughly dried and inspected for any lesions.

CURRENT RECOMMENDATIONS
Prevention of Laminitis

As an intervention to help prevent the development of laminitis, cryotherapy should be initiated during the developmental phase of laminitis and should remain applied for the duration of this phase. Horses at risk for the development of laminitis and horses with signs consistent with endotoxemia and/or SIRS should be identified and cryotherapy initiated early in treatment. Continuous digital cryotherapy is likely to produce the best results, and general recommendations contend that cryotherapy should continue for 24 to 48 hours after the resolution of clinical or laboratory signs of inflammation.[1]

Treatment of Acute Laminitis

As an intervention for the treatment of acute laminitis, less information is available, although recent literature has supported the use of digital cryotherapy as a first-line treatment for acute laminitis associated with hyperinsulinemia in horses and has shown that application of cryotherapy even after the onset of lameness in an acute laminitis model had beneficial effects.[20,27] It is likely that the reduced metabolism induced by hypothermia may be beneficial in reducing the inflammatory and enzymatic activity present in the digit in the acute phases of laminitis. In addition, cryotherapy may provide some degree of analgesia in this phase. Previous recommendations have been to apply continuous distal limb cryotherapy to acute laminitis cases for up to 7 days after initial signs, but further research is needed.[1]

Method of Cryotherapy

Several methods are available for achieving digital cryotherapy in horses (**Fig. 1**). Current evidence recommends that hoof temperatures should be maintained lower than 10°C to achieve effective digital hypothermia. Methods that have successfully achieved this goal and have been experimentally validated include immersion of the distal limb and the entire hoof in ice and water, a prototype dry sleeve application, and a sleeve-style ice boot that does not include the hoof.[29–31] Immersion of the distal limb and hoof can be achieved by applying wader-style ice boots or using empty fluid bags filled with ice and water: both of these methods were found to maintain hoof wall surface temperatures less than 5°C.[31] One study found that ice slurry bags using 5-L fluid bags containing an ice slurry, as well as wader boot methods, produced similar digital cooling, and proposed that this fluid bag method may be a readily available and practical method for cryotherapy in horses.[32] Methods that did not maintain hoof surface temperatures less than 10°C included dry application of ice packs to the hoof and/or distal limb, as well as a commercially available ice boot that incorporated the distal limb but not the hoof (Jack's Boots, Jack's Inc, Washington, OH, USA).[31] However, Burke and colleagues[29] evaluated the Jack's commercially available sleeve-style ice boot that does not incorporate the hoof in healthy horses and horses receiving intravenous endotoxin. The boots decreased skin temperature to a mean of 7.2°C (healthy horses) and 5.8°C (endotoxemic horses) and lamellar temperature to a mean of 10.8°C (healthy horses) and 9.6°C (endotoxemic horses). The skin and lamellar temperatures were lower in endotoxemic horses than healthy horses, suggesting that significant decreases in lamellar temperature could be achieved by cooling of blood as it travels to the foot.

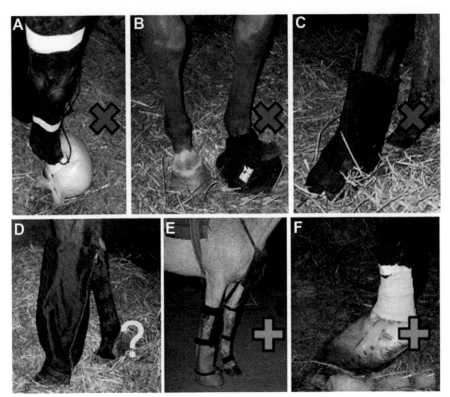

Fig. 1. Various methods of cooling the hoof. (*A*) Coronet sleeve; (*B*) ice pack (foot only); (*C*) ice pack (foot and distal limb); (*D*) commercially available ice boot; (*E*) wader-style ice boot (foot and distal limb); (*F*) fluid bag with ice. X, current research does not support this method; +, current research supports this method; ?, conflicting research. (*Adapted from* van Eps AW, Orsini JA. A comparison of seven methods for continuous therapeutic cooling of the equine digit. *Equine Vet J* 2016;48:120-124. Reprinted with permission of Andrew van Eps.)

In general, dry applications have been found to be ineffective at achieving appropriate hypothermia in the distal limb, except for a more recently evaluated prototype dry application.[30] A novel dry method for cryotherapy has been evaluated, using a commercially available rubber and rubber-welded fabric ice boot with cold therapy packs secured at the foot and pastern (**Fig. 2**). Hoof wall surface temperature in that study reached a minimum median temperature of 6.75°C at 68 minutes after application, suggesting this method may be an effective alternative for cryotherapy.[30]

Regardless of the method used, close monitoring for dermal injury in horses is indicated, particularly with prolonged duration of use and with sleeve-style methods involving direct contact of the skin with ice water slurries.

Best Cryotherapy Methods

Digital cryotherapy is currently one of the best therapeutic interventions available to veterinarians to help prevent the development of laminitis and to potentially help treat acute laminitis in the early stages. Based on the currently available literature, use of one of the following options is likely to achieve and maintain hoof wall temperatures below the targeted 10°C: immersion of the entire hoof and a portion of the distal

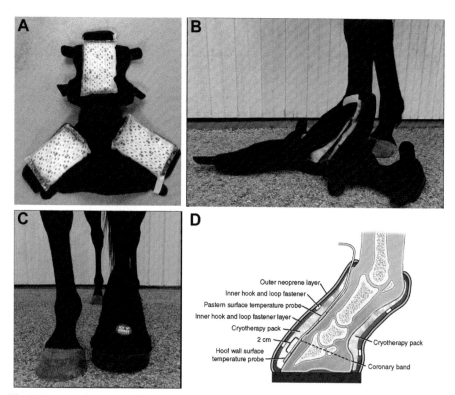

Fig. 2. Dry cryotherapy application method using a commercially available boot that encompasses the foot and pastern. Three malleable cryotherapy packs are attached directly to the internal surface of the internal loop-and-hook fastener layer (*A*). The packs and internal hook-and-loop fastener layer are then molded to the hoof and pastern to incorporate the distal limb (*B*). The boot is then secured with the outer elastic layer with hook-and-loop fastener flaps (*C*). Sagittal cut of distal limb demonstrating the arrangement of cryotherapy packs, temperature probes, and inner hook-and-loop fasteners secured (*D*). (*From* Morgan J, Stefanovski D, Lenfest M, Chatterjee S, Orsini J. Novel dry cryotherapy system for cooling the equine digit. *Vet Rec Open* 2018;5:e000244.)

limb in ice and water; a sleeve-style ice boot that does not incorporate the foot; and a prototype dry sleeve application.[2]

SUMMARY

Studies support the use of continuous digital cryotherapy for the prevention and treatment of sepsis-related and hyperinsulinemic laminitis, reducing the severity of lesions in experimental models, and reducing the incidence of laminitis in clinical cases. Digital hypothermia should be a standard of care for both prevention of laminitis and treatment of the acute phases of laminitis, as it is currently the best therapeutic intervention available to veterinarians to help prevent development of laminitis and to help treatment of acute laminitis in the early stages. Current methods supported by the literature include the use of immersion of the entire hoof and a portion of the distal limb in ice and water, a sleeve-style ice boot that does not incorporate the foot, and a prototype dry sleeve application. Distal limbs should be monitored closely for potential adverse effects.

CLINICS CARE POINTS

- Use digital hypothermia to help prevent the development of laminitis in sepsis-related conditions, as well as in the early phases of treatment of acute endocrinopathic laminitis.
- Maintain hoof temperatures less than 10°C for effective digital hypothermia. Currently available options include the following:
  - Immersion of the distal limb and entire hoof in ice and water
  - Sleeve-style ice boot
  - Prototype dry sleeve application
- Avoid dry application of ice packs to the hoof and/or distal limb.
- Monitor distal limbs closely for dermal injury in horses where prolonged cryotherapy is used.

DISCLOSURE

There are no conflicts of interest to disclose.

REFERENCES

1. van Eps AW. Therapeutic hypothermia (cryotherapy) to prevent and treat acute laminitis. Vet Clin North Am Equine Pract 2010;26:125–33.
2. Bamford NJ. Clinical insights: treatment of laminitis. Equine Vet J 2019;51:145–6.
3. Cooper SM, Dawber RP. The history of cryosurgery. J R Soc Med 2001;94:196–201.
4. Swenson C, Swärd L, Karlsson J. Cryotherapy in sports medicine. Scand J Med Sci Sports 1996;6:193–200.
5. Ivers T. Cryotherapy: an in-depth study. Equine Pract 1987;9:17–9.
6. Worster AA, Gaughan EM, Hoskinson JJ, et al. Effects of external thermal manipulation on laminar temperature and perfusion scintigraphy of the equine digit. N Z Vet J 2000;48:111–6.
7. Pollitt CC, Eps AW. Prolonged, continuous distal limb cryotherapy in the horse. Equine Vet J 2004;36:216–20.
8. Douglas W, Malcolm J. The effect of localized cooling on mammalian muscle spindles. J Physiol 1955;130:53–71.
9. Webster CM, Kelly S, Koike MA, et al. Inflammation and NFκB activation is decreased by hypothermia following global cerebral ischemia. Neurobiol Dis 2009;33:301–12.
10. Scumpia PO, Sarcia PJ, Kelly KM, et al. Hypothermia induces anti-inflammatory cytokines and inhibits nitric oxide and myeloperoxidase-mediated damage in the hearts of endotoxemic rats. Chest 2004;125:1483–91.
11. Prandini MN, Neves Filho A, Lapa AJ, et al. Mild hypothermia reduces polymorphonuclear leukocytes infiltration in induced brain inflammation. Arq Neuropsiquiatr 2005;63:779–84.
12. Lim C-M, Sun Kim M, Ahn J-J, et al. Hypothermia protects against endotoxin-induced acute lung injury in rats. Intensive Care Med 2003;29:453–9.
13. Fuhrman GJ, Fuhrman FA. Oxygen consumption of animals and tissues as a function of temperature. J Gen Physiol 1959;42:715–22.
14. Palmer C, Vannucci RC, Christensen MA, et al. Regional cerebral blood flow and glucose utilization during hypothermia in newborn dogs. Anesthesiology 1989;71:730–7.

15. Polderman KH. Mechanisms of action, physiological effects, and complications of hypothermia. Crit Care Med 2009;37:186–202.
16. McGuire DA, Hendricks SD. Incidences of frostbite in arthroscopic knee surgery postoperative cryotherapy rehabilitation. Arthroscopy 2006;22:1141e1–6.
17. Ungley CC, Channell G, Richards R. The immersion foot syndrome. Wilderness Environ Med 2003;14:135–41.
18. Asplin KE, Sillence MN, Pollitt CC, et al. Induction of laminitis by prolonged hyperinsulinaemia in clinically normal ponies. Vet J 2007;174:530–5.
19. Eps AW, Pollitt CC. Equine laminitis: cryotherapy reduces the severity of the acute lesion. Equine Vet J 2004;36:255–60.
20. van Eps AW, Pollitt CC. Equine laminitis model: cryotherapy reduces the severity of lesions evaluated seven days after induction with oligofructose. Equine Vet J 2009;41:741–6.
21. van Eps AW, Pollitt CC, Underwood C, et al. Continuous digital hypothermia initiated after the onset of lameness prevents lamellar failure in the oligofructose laminitis model. Equine Vet J 2014;46:625–30.
22. Kullmann A, Holcombe SJ, Hurcombe SD, et al. Prophylactic digital cryotherapy is associated with decreased incidence of laminitis in horses diagnosed with colitis. Equine Vet J 2014;46:554–9.
23. van Eps AW, Leise BS, Watts M, et al. Digital hypothermia inhibits early lamellar inflammatory signalling in the oligofructose laminitis model. Equine Vet J 2012;44:230–7.
24. Dern K, Watts M, Werle B, et al. Effect of delayed digital hypothermia on lamellar inflammatory signaling in the oligofructose laminitis model. J Vet Intern Med 2017;31:575–81.
25. Dern K, van Eps A, Wittum T, et al. Effect of continuous digital hypothermia on lamellar inflammatory signaling when applied at a clinically-relevant timepoint in the oligofructose laminitis model. J Vet Intern Mei 2018;32:450–8.
26. Stokes SM, Belknap JK, Engiles JB, et al. Continuous digital hypothermia prevents lamellar failure in the euglycaemic hyperinsulinaemic clamp model of equine laminitis. Equine Vet J 2019;51:658–64.
27. Stokes SM, Burns TA, Watts MR, et al. Effect of digital hypothermia on lamellar inflammatory signaling in the euglycemic hyperinsulinemic clamp laminitis model. J Vet Intern Med 2020;34:1606–13.
28. Proctor-Brown L, Hicks R, Colmer S, et al. Distal limb pathologic conditions in horses treated with sleeve-style digital cryotherapy (285 cases). Res Vet Sci 2018;121:12–7.
29. Burke MJ, Tomlinson JE, Blikslager AT, et al. Evaluation of digital cryotherapy using a commercially available sleeve style ice boot in healthy horses and horses receiving I.V. endotoxin. Equine Vet J 2018;50:848–53.
30. Morgan J, Stefanovski D, Lenfest M, et al. Novel dry cryotherapy system for cooling the equine digit. Vet Rec Open 2018;5:e000244.
31. van Eps AW, Orsini JA. A comparison of seven methods for continuous therapeutic cooling of the equine digit. Equine Vet J 2016;48:120–4.
32. Reesink HL, Divers TJ, Bookbinder LC, et al. Measurement of digital laminar and venous temperatures as a means of comparing three methods of topically applied cold treatment for digits of horses. Am J Vet Res 2012;73:860–6.

Other Clinical Problems of the Equine Foot

Anton E. Fürst, Dr med vet[a],*, Christoph J. Lischer, Dr med vet[b]

KEYWORDS

- Horse • Keratoma • Foot abscess • Fracture • Navicular syndrome
- Tendon and ligament injuries • Pedal osteitis • White line disease

KEY POINTS

- The hooves bear the entire weight of the horse, and thus even minor problems have a lasting effect on performance: the adage "no hoof, no horse" remains relevant.
- MRI and CT are often the tools of choice for diagnosing hoof diseases at equine referral clinics.
- Advanced intraoperative imaging and targeted lag screw fixation substantially improve the prognosis of most fractures within the hoof capsule.
- The key for successful therapy for any disorder of the horn capsule is complete removal of all diseased and necrotic horn and maintaining hoof stability; healing takes time.
- Although hoof disorders have been a research focus for centuries, treatments that ensure return to athletic function do not exist for all problems.

INTRODUCTION

Many problems affect the equine foot. In some conditions, surgery is necessary after conservative management has failed to bring about improvement. For other problems, surgical intervention is the best or only viable treatment option. Regarding disorders of the hoof capsule, many problems have more than one predisposing cause, including poor foot hygiene; faulty feeding regimens, including vitamin and mineral deficiencies; and excessive and uncontrolled work, especially on hard and dry ground. Trimming and shoeing practices can exacerbate problems in hooves that initially had minimal change in horn quality. Fractures within the hoof capsule may involve the distal phalanx, middle phalanx, or navicular bone, and rarely all three bones concurrently. Acute trauma is the most common cause, but certain types of fractures may occur secondary to other disorders, such as osteitis or laminitis of the distal phalanx or cystlike

[a] Equine Department, Vetsuisse Faculty, University of Zurich, Winterthurerstrasse 260, Zurich 8057, Switzerland; [b] Faculty of Veterinary Medicine, Equine Clinic, Freie Universität Berlin, Oertzenweg 19b, Berlin 14163, Germany
* Corresponding author. Equine Hospital, Vetsuisse Faculty, University of Zurich, Winterthurerstrasse 260, Zurich 8057, Switzerland.
E-mail address: afuerst@vetclinics.uzh.ch

Vet Clin Equine 37 (2021) 695–721
https://doi.org/10.1016/j.cveq.2021.08.005
0749-0739/21/© 2021 Elsevier Inc. All rights reserved.

lesions in the navicular bone. Radiography allows a definitive diagnosis in most cases, but distal phalanx fractures are sometimes difficult to identify, requiring the use of computed tomography (CT) to determine the exact fracture configuration. This overview discusses frequently encountered disorders of the foot and their treatment options. Detailed information about surgical treatment is found in the reference list.[1]

KERATOMA

Although keratoma is an uncommon cause of lameness, its occurrence represents one of the most important indications for surgical invasion of the hoof capsule. Keratoma is a benign, keratin-containing, soft tissue mass that develops inside the hoof capsule. As the keratoma enlarges, pressure is generated between the hoof capsule and the distal phalanx, leading to inflammation of the corium and resorption of the underlying distal phalanx. Most keratomas manifest as an aberrant growth of keratin and are found in the dorsal, dorsolateral, or dorsomedial aspect of the wall. A spherical type of keratoma is less common and can develop anywhere in the hoof capsule[2] or even proximal to the coronary band.[3] Keratomas consist of poor-quality horn (**Fig. 1**) that quickly degenerates allowing bacteria and fungi access to the inside of the hoof wall. Therefore, keratomas are often associated with local hoof wall infections.[4]

Diagnosis
Clinical signs of keratomas include various degrees of lameness, displacement of the white line toward the sole, recurrent foot abscess, and deformation of the hoof capsule

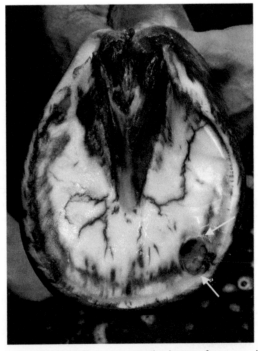

Fig. 1. A keratoma is characterized by a circumscribed area of poor-quality horn in the sole (*arrows*). Narrowing and decay of the white line is evident adjacent to the keratoma.

adjacent to the underlying keratoma.[5] Radiographically, a circular lytic area in the distal phalanx may be evident (**Fig. 2**), which should not be mistaken for the naturally occurring crena marginalis at the dorsal aspect of the distal margin of the third phalanx. Advanced three-dimensional imaging modalities, such as CT (**Fig. 3**) and MRI (**Fig. 4**), are recommended for better preoperative planning.[5–7]

Treatment and Aftercare

Successful treatment that prevents recurrence requires complete keratoma removal to its origin while maintaining the stability of the hoof capsule.[8,9] The surgery is performed with the horse under general anesthesia or standing and sedated. Successful treatment depends on complete removal of the origin of the keratoma in the stratum germinativum (**Fig. 5**). Partial removal of the hoof capsule is required and requires hoof support to maintain stability of the hoof until the wall defect has grown out.

Prognosis

Surgical treatment has a significantly better prognosis than conservative management and has been associated with a success rate of 83% compared with 43% for conservative treatment.[10] The overall prognosis for return to soundness and to the previous level of performance is very good for surgical treatment of keratomas.[5,11]

INFECTION
Hoof Abscess/Gravel

Hoof abscess is probably the most frequently diagnosed cause of severe, acute-onset lameness in equine practice. However, clinical signs may vary, and occasionally an abscess is misdiagnosed, especially when analgesics mask signs and prevent timely recognition. Common causes are sole bruise; misplacement of horseshoe nails; and penetration of the sole horn by small, pointed rocks, nails, and other foreign objects.

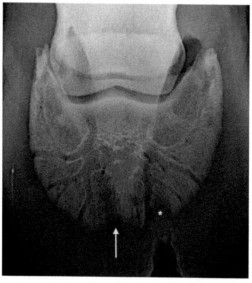

Fig. 2. Dorsopalmar radiograph of the hoof in **Fig. 1** showing a lytic area in the distal phalanx extending proximally along the hoof wall. This is a characteristic radiographic appearance of a keratoma (*asterisk*). The *arrow* is pointing to the crena marginalis.

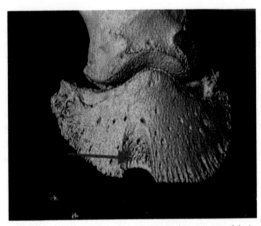

Fig. 3. Three-dimensional reconstruction of a computed tomographic image of a distal phalanx affected by a keratoma. Note the large bone defect caused by the keratoma (*arrow*).

Once bacteria or debris reach the germinal layers of the epithelium, infection ensues leading to accumulation of purulent material inside the hoof capsule (**Fig. 6**). A hoof abscess is associated with non-weight-bearing lameness because the hoof capsule provides a solid external covering with no exit route for the purulent debris; the buildup of pressure inside the hoof capsule leads to severe pain.

Diagnosis
Clinical signs include sudden severe lameness, increased warmth in the foot with a strong pulse in the distal palmar or plantar arteries, focal sensitivity to hoof testers, and occasionally an increase in rectal temperature. Soft tissue swelling in the pastern region and sometimes further proximally may be observed in long-standing cases. Local perineural anesthetic blocks aid in localizing the problem, allowing subsequent pain-free treatment. The exact location of the abscess is determined using hoof testers, although this may be hindered by the presence of thick or hard sole horn. In those cases, a suitable poultice should be applied to the foot daily to soften the hoof horn and eventually a tract may become noticeable. In some cases, radiography supports a tentative diagnosis of hoof abscess (**Fig. 7**).

Treatment and aftercare
The most important aspect of treatment is establishing a drainage route for the purulent material. The undermined and necrotic horn is carefully removed, and the infected

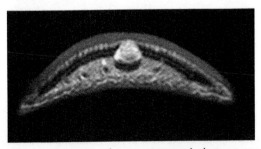

Fig. 4. MRI (T2-weighted turbo spin echo tra sequence) shows a space-occupying mass causing a defect in the distal phalanx and an indentation of the dermal/epidermal laminae.

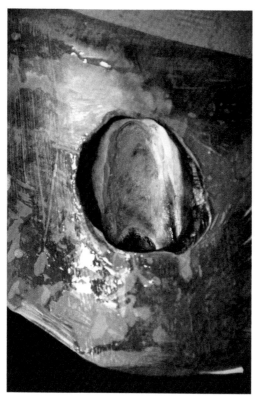

Fig. 5. Postoperative appearance after removal of a keratoma through a circular window in the hoof wall. All soft tissue adjacent to the keratoma was resected exposing the distal phalanx.

area is cleaned with disinfectant solution and covered with a gauze sponge soaked in an antiseptic solution and a hoof bandage. The bandage is changed after 2 to 3 days, at which time the defect is thoroughly examined, and any additional undermined horn carefully removed. Once the site is dry, the horse is reshod. Antimicrobial therapy is only indicated when involvement of deeper structures is suspected.

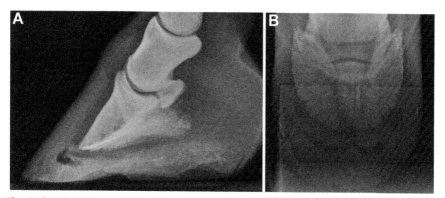

Fig. 6. (*A, B*). Lateromedial and dorsoproximal radiographs showing gas or fluid pockets indicative of a large hoof abscess.

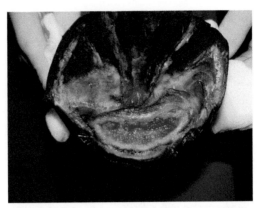

Fig. 7. The same hoof abscess shown in **Fig. 6**, 3 weeks after it was diagnosed radiographically. All undermined and necrotic horn was removed and the hoof was bandaged. Antimicrobials were not given.

Prognosis

Generally, the prognosis for uncomplicated solar abscesses is good.[12] If the abscess is left untreated or is not managed properly, the infection can migrate under the sole or along the wall away from the sole-wall junction and even break through at the coronary band (**Fig. 8**). Advanced abscesses can take weeks to heal completely,[4] especially if a substantial amount of hoof wall needs to be resected (**Fig. 9**). Extension of the infection into the distal phalanx or the distal interphalangeal (DIP) joint (**Fig. 10**) is uncommon.[12]

Septic Osteitis

Septic pedal osteitis is the result of a hoof abscess that becomes chronic and extends into the distal phalanx.[13,14] Comprehensive radiographic evaluation with or without a probe inserted into the draining tract may be diagnostic because radiographic changes in the distal phalanx become visible at this stage of infection. Sequestration of bone is a common sequela of septic pedal osteitis. If radiographs are inconclusive, three-dimensional imaging, such as CT, cone-beam CT, or MRI, is indicated.[15]

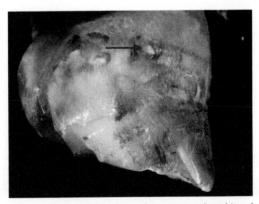

Fig. 8. Purulent material (*arrow*) draining from the coronary band in a horse with a chronic hoof abscess. The region proximal to the coronary band is markedly swollen.

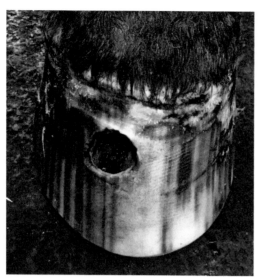

Fig. 9. A chronic hoof abscess that required fenestration of the hoof wall.

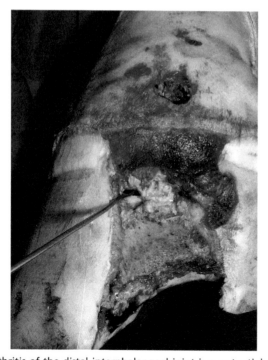

Fig. 10. Septic arthritis of the distal interphalangeal joint is a potential complication of a hoof abscess. The image shows the postoperative results of an abscess proximal to the coronary band that was drained and flushed and curettage of the affected bone. A metal probe has been inserted into the distal interphalangeal joint space.

Treatment consists of surgical debridement of the infected bone or removal of the sequestrum. In most cases, the draining tract is followed to the site of osteitis. It is important to remove all loose horn and affected soft tissue around the fistula. In cases where the infection has extended along the side wall, all of the undermined wall must be carefully removed until normal wall is present. The exposed necrotic and infected bone must be curetted aggressively until healthy bone is reached. Systemic and local antibiotic therapy is indicated. Orthopedic shoeing, to maintain stability of the hoof capsule, is crucial to the prevention of laminitis in the support/contralateral limb.

Solar Penetration

Etiology

Superficial solar penetration of the equine hoof is readily treated with conservative management. However, puncture of the solar surface of the hoof by nails or other sharp objects, such as screws or pieces of wire, have the potential to involve important structures. These wounds may appear small, but they are often deep and can have disastrous effects when such structures as the distal phalanx, distal sesamoid bone (DSB), DIP joint, navicular bursa, deep digital flexor tendon (DDFT), or tendon sheath are penetrated (**Fig. 11**).[16,17] Furthermore, the penetrating object is often contaminated with soil, rust, or manure, which can lead to a serious infection, because the superficial wound in the sole usually seals quickly, leaving little or no area for drainage.

Depending on the location, deep puncture wounds are extremely serious and difficult to treat, and affected horses are often referred to specialized clinics for surgical treatment.[18] For these reasons, deep puncture wounds must be treated as an

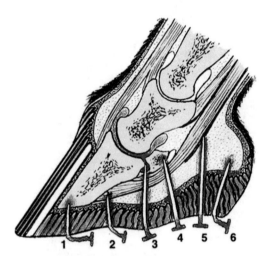

Fig. 11. Depending on the site of entry of a sharp foreign body into the foot, different anatomic structures may be affected. From dorsal to palmar/plantar: distal phalanx at the toe (1); insertion of the deep digital flexor tendon at the level of the dorsal third of the frog (2); deep digital flexor tendon, impar ligament, and possibly distal interphalangeal joint at the level of the middle of the frog (3); deep digital flexor tendon, distal sesamoid bone, and navicular bursa at the level of the palmar/plantar third of the frog (4); hoof cushion, deep digital flexor tendon, and tendon sheath at the level of the palmar/plantar aspect of the frog (5); and hoof cushion at the level of the palmar/plantar-most part of the frog (6).

emergency to establish a definite diagnosis and prevent the infection of bones, joints, and other synovial structures.

Emergency management

Ideally, radiographic images should be taken before the penetrating object is removed but when this is not feasible, the nail or foreign body should be promptly removed. However, it is imperative to note the depth and direction of the tract and mark the point of entry on the sole or record it on a photograph because it rapidly becomes inapparent. The point of entry is cleaned, and the entire hoof is bandaged. With suspected or confirmed injury to deeper structures, such as the navicular bursa, DIP joint, the digital flexor tendon sheath, or the DDFT, the horse must be referred immediately for surgical treatment under general anesthesia, where flushing of synovial structures or debridement of the DDFT is done.

A definite diagnosis is based on identification of the puncture tract. Subsequently, the sole is aseptically prepared, a sterile metal probe is inserted, and the hoof is radiographed in two planes to demonstrate the direction and the depth of the tract (**Fig. 12**). Injection of contrast material into the navicular bursa, the DIP joint, and the digital flexor tendon sheath independently, may determine the integrity of the synovial membrane (**Fig. 13**). However, these techniques are not reliable for assessing soft tissue injury other than synovial structures.[19] There is growing evidence that a combined approach using MRI, radiography, and synoviocentesis is optimal for identifying the structures affected, assisting in selection of the most effective surgical approach, and prognosticating.[19,20]

Treatment

The classical street nail procedure is still used with good success (**Fig. 14**),[1] especially when infected tendons and bone are identified. Endoscopic lavage with curettage of the puncture wound tract from the solar aspect has been successfully used for treatment of contaminated or septic navicular bursae. It permits a less-invasive approach

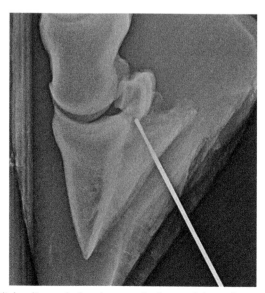

Fig. 12. Lateromedial radiograph showing a probe inserted through a puncture wound that extended into the navicular bursa and distal sesamoid bone.

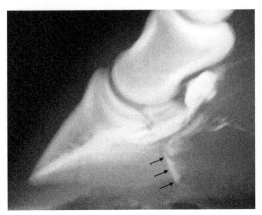

Fig. 13. Lateromedial radiographic contrast study of the navicular bursa showing contrast media (*arrows*) exiting through the puncture wound.

to the penetrated structures and allows debridement to be carried out under endoscopic guidance.[21,22]

Prognosis

Penetrating injuries located centrally in the foot without involvement of synovial structures have a favorable prognosis.[23] The postoperative prognosis for solar foot penetration with synovial involvement is fair to guarded (56%) for survival-to-discharge and poor (29%–36%) for return to preinjury athletic function.[17,23,24] In a recent study, 16 of 19 horses (84%) returned to their previous level of use after navicular bursotomy (street nail procedure) for treatment of a septic/contaminated bursa.[25] A poor outcome in horses with synovial sepsis following solar foot penetration is likely to be multifactorial, but a longer interval between injury and treatment is one of the most important factors for failure to return to preoperative level of performance.

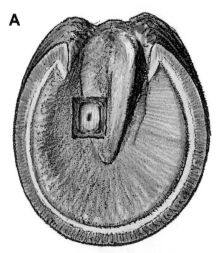
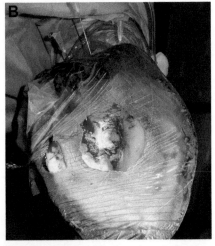

Fig. 14. Illustration (*A*) and intraoperative view (*B*) of a "street nail procedure." The deep digital flexor tendon has been fenestrated and the flexural surface of the navicular bone is visible.

FRACTURES

Fractures within the hoof capsule may occur in the distal phalanx, middle phalanx, or navicular bone, and rarely are all three bones concurrently affected. Acute trauma is the most common cause, but certain types of fractures may occur secondary to other conditions, such as osteitis and laminitis of the distal phalanx or cystlike lesions in the navicular bone. The most common cause is fast or excessive work,[26] but trauma sustained during a kick to a hard, nonmovable object and laceration of the hoof capsule may result in fractures.

The most common clinical presentation is a moderate to severe lameness that is exacerbated during turns and becomes worse within 24 hours of injury. Resolution of clinical signs is achieved with regional anesthesia of the distal phalangeal region. Hoof abscess should be considered in the differential diagnosis.

Fracture of the Distal Phalanx

Fractures of the distal phalanx occur in horses of all ages, even in young foals.[27,28] They are traditionally classified into six types (**Fig. 15**). A nonarticular fracture involving the solar margins of the palmar/plantar process in foals has been added to the system as type VII.[29] Some complicated fractures involve several fracture types and therefore cannot be classified as one type.[26,30]

   I. Abaxial/paramedian fractures without joint involvement
  II. Abaxial/paramedian fractures with joint involvement
 III. Axial and periaxial fractures with joint involvement
 IV. Fractures of the extensor process
  V. Multifragment (comminuted) fractures with joint involvement
 VI. Solar margin fractures

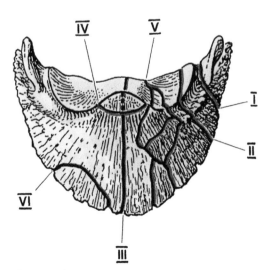

Fig. 15. Illustration showing the classification of distal phalangeal fractures in horses: I, abaxial nonarticular fracture; II, abaxial articular fracture; III, axial and periaxial articular fracture; IV, extensor process fracture; V, multifragment articular fracture; and VI, solar margin fracture.

Diagnosis

In most cases, standard radiographic views (lateromedial, dorsopalmar/dorsoplantar, and dorso65°proximal-palmaro-/plantarodistal oblique) confirm the diagnosis, although minimal displacement of the fracture occasionally makes this difficult. Additionally, the irregular border of the distal phalanx and debris attached to the hoof capsule can interfere with identification of a fracture line.[31] It is important to distinguish vascular channels from fractures. The presence of thin lines crossing vascular channels at different angles indicates a fracture. Abaxial type I and II fractures are particularly difficult to recognize on standard projections because they are usually only minimally displaced. Additional oblique radiographic views, such as dorsal45°proximal45°lateral-palmaro-/plantarodistal oblique, palmar/plantar45°proximal45°lateral-dorsodistal oblique, and palmaro-/plantaroproximal-palmaro-/plantarodistal oblique radiographic views, are recommended in this situation.

When no fractures are identified, the horse should be kept in a box stall and radiographic examination repeated 7 to 10 days later.[32] With time, displacement of the fracture and osteolysis at the fracture margins result in enlargement of the fracture gap, which facilitates identification of the fracture. CT and MRI provide the best delineation of the fracture configuration and are especially useful for assessment of articular fractures of the distal phalanx.[32–34]

Treatment

Some fractures of the distal phalanx are managed conservatively with stall rest and hoof immobilization using a foot cast or orthopedic shoeing. Surgical options include arthroscopic removal of intra-articular fragments and internal fixation. A lag screw fixation technique should be considered for intra-articular fractures (types II, III, IV, and V) because fracture compression provides stability and decreases the articular fracture gap that remains with conservative treatment. Foals (up to 1 year) are best treated with stall rest.[28,35]

Abaxial Fractures Without Joint Involvement (Type I)

Nonarticular fractures are managed conservatively using a fiberglass cast around the hoof capsule to provide support for 2 months. The sole region must be filled with a silicone or polyurethane pad to impede movement of the hoof capsule. Alternatively, a bar shoe with large side clips combined with a full pad is applied to support the heels and to limit hoof expansion during loading (**Fig. 16**). Stall rest, for approximately 2 months, is required. Follow-up radiographs are taken to evaluate fracture healing and to identify fracture displacement.

Usually after 4 months, the horse is ridden at a walk on level ground using regular shoes. The workload is gradually increased according to comfort level. This type of fracture has a good prognosis for return to athletic function.[36] It generally takes 4 to 6 months for the fracture to heal. However, radiographically the fracture line is visible for much longer. Initially a fibrous union develops, which ossifies at 6 to 12 months. In some cases, delayed malunion or nonunion develops.

Axial, Periaxial, and Abaxial Fractures with Joint Involvement (Types II and III)

Intra-articular fractures may be managed with stall rest and hoof immobilization or surgically using a lag screw technique, but there is ongoing debate as to whether surgical treatment as first reported by Sonnichsen[37] and Pettersson[38] is superior to conservative management. A recent retrospective analysis of 96 type II and III fractures did not find a difference in outcome between conservative and surgical management.[36]

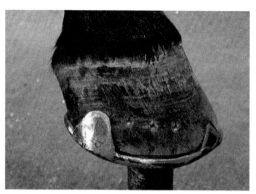

Fig. 16. A bar shoe with large side clips and a full pad limits hoof expansion during loading. This shoe is recommended for conservative management of distal phalanx fractures.

However, many cases in that study were operated without adequate intraoperative imaging techniques.

In principle, optimal healing of simple fractures is achieved when the fracture is stabilized and compressed using lag screw fixation technique. Although conceptually simple, internal fixation of the distal phalanx remains challenging, especially for type II fractures, because screw placement deep within the hoof wall has an extremely narrow anatomic margin for error.[3,39] Surgical repair has been accomplished with the aid of two-dimensional imaging techniques, but recent reports have demonstrated the superiority and simplicity of three-dimensional imaging for preoperative planning, intraoperative control, and postoperative evaluation.[39]

Conservative management of articular fractures requires stall rest for a minimum of 4 months. This is followed by 2 months of hand-walking and an additional 2 months of exercise under saddle at a walk. The prognosis for return to athletic function is guarded in horses older than 3 years, but is good in horses younger than 2 years.[38,40] Frequently, delayed union, malunion, or nonunion (**Fig. 17**) associated with osteoarthritis and chronic lameness is seen after conservative therapy.[39]

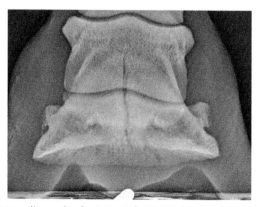

Fig. 17. Dorsopalmar radiograph of a type III fracture of the distal phalanx 2.5 years after fracture occurrence. This horse was treated conservatively and the fracture line is still clearly visible.

Several experimental and clinical studies have shown that screw fixation of the distal phalanx using a lag technique improved fracture reduction and stabilization, which hastens fracture healing and likely reduces development of osteoarthritis of the DIP joint.[39,41,42] The authors of this article are convinced that surgical treatment with one or two cortical screws inserted in lag fashion substantially improves the prognosis of these fractures. However, the position of the screws is crucial and the use of advanced imaging techniques is mandatory. In most type II and III fractures, a single 4.5-mm cortical screw inserted in lag fashion creates sufficient compression and stabilization (**Fig. 18**).

Postoperative care entails stall rest for 2 months followed by hand-walking for 2 more months. Fracture healing is expected 6 to 10 months postoperatively. Screws are left in place unless there are complications, such as postoperative infection and abscess formation around the screw head. In these cases, screw removal is required to resolve the infection.

Extensor Process Fragments (Type IV)

The etiopathogenesis of extensor process fragments includes hyperextension injury or avulsion injury (fragment pulled away by the extensor tendon). In many horses, fragmentation of the extensor process is an incidental radiographic finding in the absence of clinical signs. They are usually removed as a preventive measure because they are mobile and in contact with the articular surfaces.[43] Osteochondral fragments in the dorsal pouch of the DIP joint associated with lameness should be evaluated carefully and if the cause of lameness is localized to the DIP joint, arthroscopic removal is strongly recommended. Fragment removal is accomplished by routine arthroscopy. The short-term prognosis for resolution of lameness is good, but a more guarded prognosis for long-term soundness has been reported.[44]

Large fragments should be stabilized with a 3.5- or 4.5-mm cortex screw inserted in lag fashion (**Fig. 19**) because conservative treatment is often associated with complications, such as dislocation of the fragment and nonunion.[45,46] Postoperatively, a cast including the foot or the distal limb should be applied.

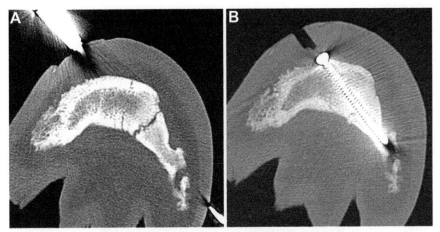

Fig. 18. Surgical treatment of a type II fracture of the distal phalanx using intraoperative computed tomography. (*A*) The correct position of the aiming device is confirmed before drilling the glide hole through the hoof capsule. (*B*) Stabilization of the fracture with one 4.5-mm cortex screw in lag fashion. Note the obvious interfragmentary compression.

Arthroscopic removal of large fragments that occupy more than 25% of the surface of the DIP joint has been achieved successfully in Friesian horses.[45] The long-term outcome was good, and remodeling of the remaining extensor process and new subchondral bone were often observed in horses with functional recovery.

Multifragment Fractures (Type V)

Multifragment fractures are always accompanied by severe lameness. Radiographically, several fracture lines are seen, but three-dimensional imaging is required to fully understand the fracture configuration (**Fig. 20**). Internal fixation with cortical screws inserted in lag fashion should be attempted when there is a chance to reconstruct and stabilize the DIP joint (**Fig. 21**).

Solar Margin Fractures (Type VI)

Solar margin fractures occur often and are frequently misdiagnosed.[31,47] A recent study showed a high prevalence in young Thoroughbred foals.[29] Direct or blunt trauma, which may occur when the horse kicks a hard, immobile object, is a common cause of solar margin fractures. These fractures can also develop as a result of chronic laminitis. Most solar margin fractures heal by bony union, and resorption of small fragments may occur. Surgical removal of fragments has been described in individual cases, especially when infection develops.

Fractures of the Distal Sesamoid Bone

Fractures of the DSB (navicular bone) are uncommon. They are diagnosed more often in thoracic limbs than in pelvic limbs and are classified as avulsion or chip fractures, simple fractures of the body, comminuted fractures, and frontal fractures.[48]

Avulsion fractures of the distal margin (distal border fragments) usually correspond with a concave fracture bed at the distal border of the navicular bone. Although they commonly present with other radiographic changes consistent with navicular bone pathology, the pathogenesis is still poorly understood, and their clinical relevance remains unclear.[49] Most of the simple fractures occur abaxially in a vertical or slightly oblique direction (**Fig. 22**) with a varying degree of displacement. Multifragment fractures are uncommon and, in most cases, carry a poor prognosis. Fractures in the frontal plane are highly unusual. Most fractures of the DSB are associated with trauma and result from excessive or repetitive loading through the middle and distal phalanges

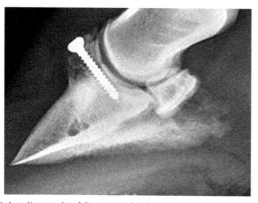

Fig. 19. Lateromedial radiograph of fixation of a fractured extensor process using a 4.5-mm lag screw in lag fashion. This radiograph was taken 2 days after surgery.

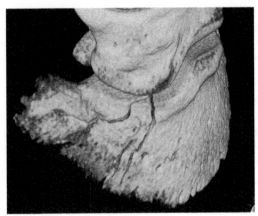

Fig. 20. Three-dimensional computed tomography is indispensable for fully understanding the configuration of a multifragment fracture of the pedal bone.

and the DDFT. Occasionally, a preexisting pathologic condition in the DSB predisposes it to fracture. In these cases, chronic navicular disease is usually implicated.[50]

All standard radiographic views of the DSB should be taken (lateromedial, upright pedal, skyline) to rule out the potential presence of a bipartite or tripartite DSB (two or three ossification centers) or other disorders. Air shadows of the sulci of the frog

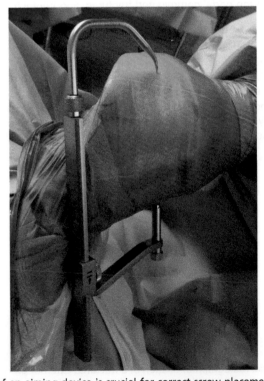

Fig. 21. The use of an aiming device is crucial for correct screw placement.

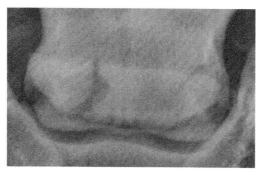

Fig. 22. Dorsopalmar radiograph of a fracture of the navicular bone shows complete nonunion of the fracture 8 months after the injury.

project over the DSB and is mistaken for fracture lines. Therefore, it is important to pack the sulci with a suitable modeling compound before taking the radiographs.

Conservative management includes stall rest and remedial shoeing to immobilize the hoof capsule (quarter clips and frog support) and to elevate the heel (wedge) for a minimum of 4 months. This is followed by small paddock exercise and use of a shoe with thick (reinforced) branches.[51] Even if the patient improves clinically during the first few months, in most cases an osseous union cannot be detected radiographically (**Fig. 23**). Healing requires 10 to 12 months, but it is generally accepted that the prognosis for conservative management is guarded to poor for return to athletic function.[52] Therefore, it is reasonable to use cortical screws inserted in lag fashion to achieve interfragmentary compression and to promote bone healing. However, the difficulty lies in correct placement of the screw and in avoiding penetration of the DIP joint and the navicular bursa. This procedure should be reserved for specialized equine hospitals because a suitable aiming device and fluoroscopy are mandatory for proper screw placement. Further improvement of accuracy in screw placement

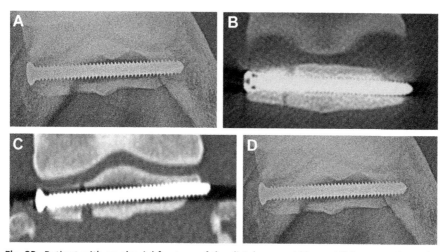

Fig. 23. Patient with an abaxial fracture of the distal sesamoid bone (*A*) Preoperative radiograph. (*B,C*) Intraoperative computed tomographic study showing fixation with a 4.0 mm cortical screw in lag fashion. (*D*) Postoperative radiograph (Courtesy F. Theis, Zurich).

is achieved with CT-guided screw insertion[41] or computer-assisted navigation.[53] The authors of this article believe that use of a 4.0-mm cortical screw inserted in lag fashion works well. Healing of fractures treated with screw fixation takes 6 to 12 months. The prognosis is guarded for return to athletic competition but is favorable in horses used for pleasure riding.[52]

NAVICULAR SYNDROME

Navicular disease or syndrome has been described as a chronic thoracic limb lameness related to pain arising from the DSB and closely related structures including the collateral suspensory ligaments of the navicular bone, the distal sesamoidean impar ligament, the navicular bursa, and the DDFT. The disease is characterized by degenerative changes in these structures, but clinicians like to use the term "palmar foot pain" or "palmar foot syndrome" to describe horses with chronic, mostly bilateral thoracic limb lameness that improves after palmar digital (PD) nerve blocks. This is a useful strategy to avoid characterizing affected horses with the syndrome provided that radiographic diagnosis is inconclusive.

MRI is the standard method for obtaining a definitive diagnosis in horses with palmar foot pain, and follow-up MRIs are extremely useful for monitoring the progression of disease and evaluating the effect of treatment.[54] The etiopathogenesis of the condition is multifactorial, and many theories have been proposed.[55–58] Vascular compromise and biomechanical abnormalities leading to tissue degeneration are the most common causes discussed. Another theory combines those two etiologies to explain the development of navicular disease/syndrome in horses.[59,60] Repetitive loading with nonphysiologic biomechanical forces combined with impaired venous drainage causes venous hypertension in the bone marrow resulting in intraosseous hypertension and bone edema. This compartment syndrome–like condition triggers the accumulation of osmotically active proteins in the subchondral bone, which is characterized by increased tissue pressure, acidosis, pain, and a vicious circle of progressive pathologic changes. The athletic activity of the horse and skeleton conformation are predisposing factors that increase biomechanical forces in the navicular apparatus. The disease is degenerative and progressive and therefore it is not surprising that middle aged horses are predominantly affected, and the condition is not curable.

Conservative Treatment

Standardized medical treatment of navicular disease/syndrome is not currently available. For this reason, management of the disorder is aimed at pain relief rather than treatment of the underlying cause. Various drugs, including acetylsalicylic acid, pentoxifylline, isoxsuprine, bisphosphonates (tiludronate, clodronate), benzopyrone, and calcium dobesilate, have been proposed, but there is no accepted clinical evidence to support the recommendation of one over another. Bisphosphonates are widely used in horses to control clinical signs associated with navicular disease. Tiludronate and clodronate were approved by the Food and Drug Administration for the treatment of navicular disease. Double-blinded, placebo-controlled, clinical trials[61,62] provided subjective evidence that each of these drugs is efficacious at the approved dose and route of administration as an adjunct treatment of navicular disease/syndrome. Further studies are needed to determine the true efficacy of bisphosphonates in horses with navicular disease/syndrome. Standard management strategies include rest and controlled exercise, remedial shoeing, and intrasynovial medication. Nonsteroidal anti-inflammatory drugs are used as the first-line treatment or when the horse is severely lame.

Multiple shoeing methods have been proposed, but there is no single shoe type that is effective in all horses with navicular disease/syndrome. However, the following goals for trimming and shoeing are widely accepted[63]: (1) restore normal foot balance; (2) correct foot problems in the palmar aspect of the hoof, such as underrun or contracted heels and sheared quarters/heels; (3) reduce biomechanical forces on the navicular region; (4) ease break-over at the toe; and (5) support heels and prevent heel descent during loading.

Injection of various medications into the DIP joint or into the navicular bursa is often used as adjunctive treatment to provide transient relief of clinical signs. Commonly used drugs include corticosteroids alone; corticosteroids with hyaluronic acid; and biologic therapies, such as autologous conditioned serum or plasma. There is no evidence of their efficacy, and thus the choice is entirely empirical. The decision to treat the synovial cavity is based on the response to synovial analgesia and the results of imaging studies.

Surgical Management

Surgery is usually reserved for cases of navicular disease/syndrome that have not responded to conservative management. Three different surgical procedures have been published in the last 20 years, but none has been associated with a long-term successful outcome: navicular suspensory desmotomy, periarterial sympathectomy, and PD neurectomy. Treatment using these surgical procedures should always be combined with remedial trimming and shoeing.

Palmar Digital Neurectomy

The most common surgical technique for elimination of lameness associated with navicular disease/syndrome is PD neurectomy. It is usually a last resort after other treatment options have failed. The prognosis after PD neurectomy seems to be good initially but becomes less favorable with time. A recent study concluded that 92% of horses had a positive response to surgery and were able to return to previous athletic use for an average of 20 months.[64] Complications associated with PD neurectomy include rupture of the DDFT, recurrence of lameness caused by reinnervation, and severe hoof infection that goes unnoticed.

COLLATERAL LIGAMENT INJURIES

Desmopathy of the collateral ligaments (CL) of the DIP joint is an important cause of foot lameness in horses. In severe cases, swelling may be palpated, eliciting a pain response, at the insertion of the middle phalanx, but often there are no localizing signs. Chronic thoracic limb lameness that varies in severity and worsens when the horse is circled is a common clinical presentation.

The medial CL of the thoracic limb is the most common site of injury, and although uncommon, the pelvic limb can also be affected. A high proportion of CL lesions of the DIP joint are located distal to the coronary band (**Fig. 24**). They require MRI (**Fig. 25**) for a definitive diagnosis and cannot be identified on ultrasound examination alone.[65] When lesions exist at the distal enthesis on the third phalanx, bony changes including cystic lesions at the site of ligament insertion are seen radiographically.

Prolonged rest and a regimented exercise program for up to 1 year and remedial trimming or shoeing are the most important aspects of conservative treatment. The aim of corrective shoeing is to decrease tension on the CL by using shoes with a wider branch on the affected side. This reduces sinking of the foot in soft ground at the expense of loading the contra-axial CL. Only one-third of cases return to full athletic

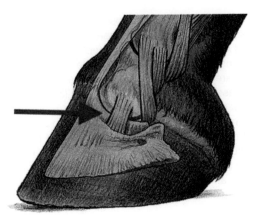

Fig. 24. Most of the collateral ligament of the distal interphalangeal joint (*arrow*) is located distal to the coronary band.

performance with conservative management, and therefore intralesional treatment with a variety of biologic agents has been suggested. There is no current evidence that this treatment is effective. Furthermore, a recent study on cadaver limbs demonstrated that successful ultrasound-guided injection into the CL and not into the joint was achieved in only 36% of the cases.[66]

DEEP DIGITAL FLEXOR TENDON LESIONS

Lesions of the DDFT are the most common soft tissue injuries of the foot and affect horses used for a wide variety of disciplines.[67,68] Advanced imaging techniques, such as MRI or CT, are required for a definitive diagnosis because clinical examination, radiography, and ultrasonography are inadequate. It is uncommon to have deep digital flexor tendinopathy alone[69] because concurrent lesions of the foot are frequently seen with MRI (**Fig. 26**). The clinical relevance of these findings is sometimes difficult to interpret. Evaluation of intrasynovial analgesia of the DIP joint and

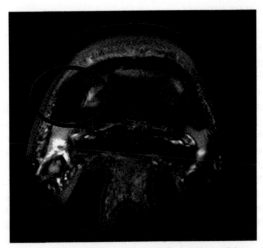

Fig. 25. MRI showing severe desmopathy of the medial collateral ligament (*circle*).

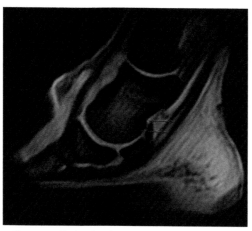

Fig. 26. MRI T2* gradient recalled echo long core lesion within the deep digital flexor tendon (*arrows*).

the navicular bursa may allow differentiation of the origin of pain. In a recent study in horses with palmar heel pain, the results of analgesia of the DIP joint and navicular bursa were significantly different 2 and 5 minutes after injection of the local anesthetic.[70]

The DDFT is bilobed within the foot and lesions may occur anywhere in the tendon from distal to the proximal interphalangeal joint to its insertion on the pedal bone. Four main types of lesions have been described: (1) core lesions, (2) dorsal border lesions, (3) sagittal plane or oblique splits, and (4) insertional lesions.[71] Lesions are most commonly seen at the level of the navicular bone and the collateral sesamoidean ligament, whereas insertional lesions are rare.[63] The etiopathogenesis of the different types of DDFF lesions is not fully understood but degenerative change as a sequel to vascular compromise and chronic repetitive trauma is most likely the underlying cause of most injuries[67] although a single traumatic event may occasionally occur.

Deep digital flexor tendinopathy in the region of the foot treated by long-term rest and 6 to 12 months of rehabilitation has a guarded to poor prognosis and is considered a career-ending injury because only a small proportion (25%–28%) of horses return to their previous level of performance.[72] Dorsal border lesions seem to have a better prognosis with 35% of horses returning to their previous level of performance and 27% remaining chronically lame. In contrast, 50% of horses with complete parasagittal split and 69% of horses with core lesions remained chronically lame.[73] The results of studies on insertional lesions, which are located in the most distal 20 mm of the DDFT and include small core lesions or sagittal plane splits, are conflicting. Two studies reported a guarded prognosis,[74,75] and one study in American quarter horse suggested that insertional lesions have a better chance of complete resolution compared with lesions located more proximally.[68]

In the last few years, other treatment options have been explored to improve the poor outcome associated with conservative management alone. However, optimal treatments tailored to address the various types of DDFT lesions in the foot have yet to be established.

Intralesional or intrasynovial administration of regenerative agents, such as autologous conditioned plasma or serum or mesenchymal stem cells, is widely used but evidence-based information about the efficacy of these treatments is lacking.

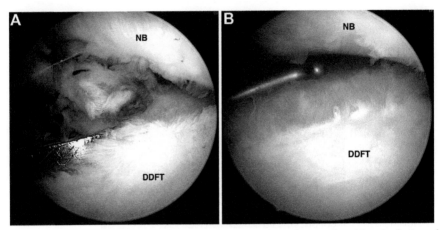

Fig. 27. (*A*) Endoscopic removal of a protruding granuloma from a dorsal border lesion of the deep digital flexor tendon in the navicular bursa. (*B*) Navicular bursa after removal of the protruding granuloma shown in A. Surgical shaver is used to debride the lesion in the deep digital flexor tendon. NB, navicular bone.

Dorsal border lesions within the (distended) navicular bursa associated with protruding granulomas (**Fig. 27**) or suspected adhesions may benefit from bursoscopy and debridement of torn tendon fibers.[76–78] Additional benefits include the opportunity to inject lesions under endoscopic guidance or, when a transthecal approach is used, to create a large open connection between the bursa and tendon sheath. This is used to ameliorate pressure within the distended bursa and to facilitate treatment of the bursa via the digital flexor tendon sheath. Other surgical options include desmotomy of the inferior check ligament of the DDFT to reduce strain on the DDFT during healing and PD neurectomy when other therapies have failed to improve lameness.[79,80] However, neurectomy is not recommended for horses with core or linear lesions because they are at greater risk of residual lameness or early recurrent lameness after surgery.[80]

SUMMARY

The equine foot is a complex biologic structure of functional significance to the integrity and well-being of the horse. A multiplicity of questions continues to drive research of this vital part of the horse anatomy. Two examples where developing concepts requires further scientific exploration and confirmation are: how exactly are impact and load forces accommodated to avoid pathologic stress and fatigue of parts; and how exactly does epidermal hoof move past the stationary dermis and distal phalanx as it grows to the ground surface, while maintaining the dermoepidermal interface. As this *Veterinary Clinics* issue title implies, the needle is moving in the right direction.

DISCLOSURE

The authors have nothing to disclose.

REFERENCES

1. Fürst A, Lischer C. Musculoskeletal system: the foot. In: Auer JA, Stick JA, Kümmerle J, et al, editors. Equine surgery. 3rd edition. St. Louis (MO): Elsevier; 2019. p. 1543–87.

2. Greet T. The management of multiple keratoma lesions in an equine foot. Equine Vet Educ 2016;28:315–8.
3. Gasiorowski JC, Getman LM, Richardson DW. Supracoronary approach for keratoma removal in horses: two cases. Equine Vet Educ 2011;23:489–93.
4. Redding WR, O'Grady SE. Nonseptic diseases associated with the hoof complex: keratoma, white line disease, canker, and neoplasia. Vet Clin North Am Equine Pract 2012;28:407–21.
5. Katzman SA, Spriet M, Galuppo LD. Outcome following computed tomographic imaging and subsequent surgical removal of keratomas in equids: 32 cases (2005-2016). J Am Vet Med Assoc 2019;254:266–74.
6. Mageed M, Elfadl A, Blum N, et al. Standing low-field magnetic resonance imaging as a diagnostic modality for solar keratoma in a horse. Equine Vet Educ 2020; 32:O56–61.
7. Sherlock C, Fairburn A, Lawson A, et al. The use of magnetic resonance imaging for the assessment of distal limb wounds in horses: a pilot study. Equine Vet Educ 2020;32:637–45.
8. Lloyd KC, Peterson PR, Wheat JD, et al. Keratomas in horses: seven cases (1975-1986). J Am Vet Med Assoc 1988;193:967–70.
9. Greet TR. Keratoma of the hoof capsule. In: Curtis S, editor. Corrective farriery. Newmarket: R&W Publications (Newmarket) Ltd; 2002. p. 171–8.
10. Bosch G, van Schie MJ, Back W. [Retrospective evaluation of surgical versus conservative treatment of keratomas in 41 lame horses (1995-2001)]. Tijdschr Diergeneeskd 2004;129:700–5.
11. Smith SJB, Clegg PD, Hughes I, et al. Complete and partial hoof wall resection for keratoma removal: post operative complications and final outcome in 26 horses (1994-2004). Equine Vet J 2006;38:127–33.
12. Cole SD, Stefanovski D, Towl S, et al. Factors associated with prolonged treatment days, increased veterinary visits and complications in horses with subsolar abscesses. Vet Rec 2019;184:251.
13. Cauvin ER, Munroe GA. Septic osteitis of the distal phalanx: findings and surgical treatment in 18 cases. Equine Vet J 1998;30:512–9.
14. Pabst B, Kaegi B. Septic osteitis of the pedal bon in horses. Pferdeheilkunde 1990;6:197–203.
15. Pauwels FE, Van der Vekens E, Christan Y, et al. Feasibility, indications, and radiographically confirmed diagnoses of standing extremity cone beam computed tomography in the horse. Vet Surg 2021;50:365–74.
16. Gibson KT, McIlwraight CW, Park RP. A radiographic study of the distal interphalangeal joint and navicular bursa of the horse. Vet Radiol 1990;31:22–5.
17. Richardson GL, O'Brien TR. Puncture wounds into the navicular bursa of the horse. Vet Radiol Ultrasound 1985;26:203–7.
18. Ludwig EK, van Harreveld PD. Equine wounds over synovial structures. Vet Clin North Am Equine Pract 2018;34:575–90.
19. de Heer N, Compagnie E, ter Braake F. Penetrating solar wounds to the foot: benefit of MRI in treatment decisions. Vlaams Diergen Tijds 2015;84:27–37.
20. Schiavo S, Cillan-Garcia E, Elce Y, et al. Horses with solar foot penetration, deep digital flexor tendon injury, and absence of concurrent synovial sepsis can have a positive outcome. Vet Radiol Ultrasound 2018;59:697–704.
21. Wright IM, Phillips TJ, Walmsley JP. Endoscopy of the navicular bursa: a new technique for the treatment of contaminated and septic bursae. Equine Vet J 1999;31:5–11.

22. Haupt JL, Caron JP. Navicular bursoscopy in the horse: a comparative study. Vet Surg 2010;39:742–7.

23. Kilcoyne I, Dechant JE, Kass PH, et al. Penetrating injuries to the frog (cuneus ungulae) and collateral sulci of the foot in equids: 63 cases (1998-2008). J Am Vet Med Assoc 2011;239:1104–9.

24. Findley JA, Pinchbeck GL, Milner PI, et al. Outcome of horses with synovial structure involvement following solar foot penetrations in four UK veterinary hospitals: 95 cases. Equine Vet J 2014;46:352–7.

25. Suarez-Fuentes DG, Caston SS, Tatarniuk DM, et al. Outcome of horses undergoing navicular bursotomy for the treatment of contaminated or septic navicular bursitis: 19 cases (2002-2016). Equine Vet J 2018;50:179–85.

26. Scott EA, Mcdole M, Shires MH. Review of 3rd phalanx fractures in the horse: 65 cases. J Am Vet Med Assoc 1979;174:1337–43.

27. Hertsch B. Zur Diagnose und Behandlung der Hufbeinfraktur. Dtsch Tierarztl Wochenschr 1972;79:517–44.

28. Yovich JV, Stashak TS, DeBowes RM, et al. Fractures of the distal phalanx of the forelimb in eight foals. J Am Vet Med Assoc 1986;189:550–4.

29. Faramarzi B, Mcmicking H, Halland S, et al. Incidence of palmar process fractures of the distal phalanx and association with front hoof conformation in foals. Equine Vet J 2015;47:675–9.

30. McDiarmid AM. An unusual case of distal phalanx fracture in a horse. Vet Rec 1995;137:613–5.

31. Honnas CM, O'Brien TR, Linford RL. Distal phalanx fractures in horses: a survey of 274 horses with radiographic assessment of healing in 36 horses. Vet Radiol 1988;29:98–107.

32. Keegan KG, Twardock AR, Losonsky JM, et al. Scintigraphic evaluation of fractures of the distal phalanx in horses: 27 cases (1979-1988). J Am Vet Med Assoc 1993;202:1993–7.

33. Martens P, Ihler CF, Rennesund J. Detection of a radiographically occult fracture of the lateral palmar process of the distal phalanx in a horse using computed tomography. Vet Radiol Ultrasound 1999;40:346–9.

34. Selberg K, Werpy N. Fractures of the distal phalanx and associated soft tissue and osseous abnormalities in 22 horses with ossified sclerotic ungual cartilages diagnosed with magnetic resonance imaging. Vet Radiol Ultrasound 2011;52:394–401.

35. Honnas CM, Vacek JR, Schumacher J. Diagnosis and treatment of articular fractures of the equine distal phalanx. Vet Med 1992;87:1208–14.

36. Rijkenhuizen AB, de Graaf K, Hak A, et al. Management and outcome of fractures of the distal phalans: a retrospective study of 285 horses with a long term outcome in 223 cases. Vet J 2012;192:176–82.

37. Sonnichsen HV. Fraktur af hovben-Kasuistik meddelelse. Nord Vet Med 1969;21:37–40.

38. Pettersson H. Conservative und surgical treatment of fractures of the third phalanx. Proc Am Ass Eq Prat 1972;18:183–92.

39. Heer C, Fürst AE, Del Chicca F, et al. Comparison of 3D-assisted surgery and conservative methods for treatment of type III fractures of the distal phalanx in horses. Equine Vet Educ 2020;32:42–51.

40. Ohlsson J, Jansson N. Conservative treatment of intra-articular distal phalanx fractures in horses not used for racing. Aust Vet J 2005;83:221–3.

41. Gasiorowski JC, Richardson DW. Clinical use of computed tomography and surface markers to assist internal fixation within the equine hoof. Vet Surg 2015;44:214–22.

42. Kay AT, Durgam S, Stewart M, et al. Effect of cortical screw diameter on reduction and stabilization of type III distal phalanx fractures: an equine cadaveric study. Vet Surg 2016;45:1025–33.

43. Boening KJ, Von Saldern FC, Leendertse IP, et al. Diagnostische und operative Arthroskopie am Hufgelenk des Pferdes. Pferdeheilkunde 1988;4:155–60.

44. Crowe OM, Hepburn RJ, Kold SE, et al. Long-term outcome after arthroscopic debridement of distal phalanx extensor process fragmentation in 13 horses. Vet Surg 2010;39:107–14.

45. Braake FT. Arthroscopic removal of large fragments of the extensor process of the distal phalanx in 4 horses. Equine Vet Educ 2005;17:101–5.

46. Haynes PF, Adams OR. Internal fixation of fractured extensor process of third phalanx in a horse. J Am Vet Med Assoc 1974;164:61–3.

47. Honnas CM, O'Brien TR, Linford RL. Solar margin fractures of the equine distal phalanx. Proc Am Assoc Equine Pract 1987;33:399–411.

48. Eichenberger S, Fürst A, Suarez Sancheez-Andrade J, et al. Avulsionsfraktur des Margo ligamenti distal am Strahlbein bei einem dreieinhalb Monate alten Fohlen. Pferdeheilkunde 2021;37:379–85.

49. Biggi M, Dyson S. Distal border fragments and shape of the navicular bone: radiological evaluation in lame horses and horses free from lameness. Equine Vet J 2012;44:325–31.

50. Hoegaerts M, Pille F, De Clercq T, et al. Comminuted fracture of the distal sesamoid bone and distal rupture of the deep digital flexor tendon. Vet Radiol Ultrasound 2005;46:234–7.

51. Hertsch B, Königsmann D. Die Sagittalfrakturen des Strahlbeines beim Pferd - ein Beitrag zur Diagnose und Therapie. Pferdeheilkunde 1993;9:3–13.

52. Lillich JD, Ruggles AJ, Gabel A, et al. Fracture of the distal sesamoid bone in horses: 17 cases (1982-1992). J Am Vet Med Assoc 1995;207:924–7.

53. Gygax D, Lischer C, Auer JA. Computer-assisted surgery for screw insertion into the distal sesamoid bone in horses: an in vitro study. Vet Surg 2006;35:626–33.

54. Janssen J, Mair T, Reardon R, et al. Effects of calcium dobesilate on horses with an increased signal intensity in the navicular bone in fat suppressed images on MRI: pilot study. Pferdeheilkunde 2011;27:601–8.

55. Dyson SJ. Navicular disease and other soft tissue causes of palmar foot pain. In: Ross MW, Dyson SJ, editors. Diagnosis and management of lameness in the horse. Philadelphia (PA): Saunders; 2003. p. 286–99.

56. Wright IM. A study of 118 cases of navicular disease: treatment by navicular suspensory desmotomy. Equine Vet J 1993;25:501–9.

57. Wright IM, Kidd L, Thorp BH. Gross, histological and histomorphometric features of the navicular bone and related structures in the horse. Equine Vet J 1998;30:220–34.

58. Rijkenhuizen AB. Navicular disease: a review of what's new. Equine Vet J 2006;38:82–8.

59. Fricker C, Bucher K, Stuker G. [Are degenerative joint diseases chronic compartment syndromes?]. Schweiz Arch Tierheilkd 1995;137:137–40.

60. Casley-Smith JR, Casley-Smith JR. High-protein oedemas and the benzo-pyrones. Sydney (Australia): J.B. Lippincott Company; 1986.

61. Denoix JM, Thibaud D, Riccio B. Tiludronate as a new therapeutic agent in the treatment of navicular disease: a double-blind placebo-controlled clinical trial. Equine Vet J 2003;35:407–13.

62. Frevel M, King BL, Kolb DS. Clodronate disodium for treatment of clinical signs of navicular disease: a double-blinded placebo-controlled clinical trial. Pferdeheilkunde 2017;33:271–9.

63. Eggleston RB, Baxter GM, Belknap J, et al. Lameness of the distal limb: navicular region/palmar foot. Adams and Stashak's Lameness in Horses 2020;439–595.

64. Gutierrez-Nibeyro SD, Werpy NM, White NA 2nd, et al. Outcome of palmar/plantar digital neurectomy in horses with foot pain evaluated with magnetic resonance imaging: 50 cases (2005-2011). Equine Vet J 2015;47:160–4.

65. Beasley B, Selberg K, Giguère S, et al. Magnetic resonance imaging characterisation of lesions within the collateral ligaments of the distal interphalangeal joint: 28 cases. Equine Vet Educ 2020;32:11–7.

66. Smith R, Parsons J, Dixon J. Risk of intra-articular injection with longitudinal ultrasound-guided injection of collateral ligaments of the equine distal interphalangeal joint. Vet Radiol Ultrasound 2020;61:67–76.

67. Blunden A, Murray R, Dyson S. Lesions of the deep digital flexor tendon in the digit: a correlative MRI and post mortem study in control and lame horses. Equine Vet J 2009;41:25–33.

68. Lutter JD, Schneider RK, Sampson SN, et al. Medical treatment of horses with deep digital flexor tendon injuries diagnosed with high-field-strength magnetic resonance imaging: 118 cases (2000-2010). J Am Vet Med Assoc 2015;247:1309–18.

69. Gutierrez-Nibeyro SD, Werpy NM, Gold SJ, et al. Standing MRI lesions of the distal interphalangeal joint and podotrochlear apparatus occur with a high frequency in warmblood horses. Vet Radiol Ultrasound 2020;61:336–45.

70. Katrinaki V, Estrada RJ, Mählmann K, et al. Use of a wireless sensor-based system to objectively evaluate the response to intra-synovial analgesia of the distal interphalangeal joint and to navicular bursa in horses with forelimb foot pain. Equine Vet J 2021.

71. Schramme M. Treatment of tendinopathy in the foot: what have we learned so far? Equine Vet Education 2018;30:545–8.

72. Schramme M. Deep digital flexor tendonopathy in the foot. Equine Vet Educ 2011;23:403–15.

73. Cillán-García E, Milner P, Talbot A, et al. Deep digital flexor tendon injury within the hoof capsule; does lesion type or location predict prognosis? Vet Rec 2013;173:70.

74. Boswell J.C. Does a DDFT injury in the foot mean the end of the horse's athletic career? In: Proceedings of the 48th British Equine Veterinary Congress. Newmarket; Equine Veterinary Journal Ltd. p 20.

75. Hewitt-Dedman C, Biggi M, Van Zadelhoff C, et al. Imaging findings and clinical outcome of foot pain attributable to insertional deep digital flexor tendon injury and/or fluid signal within the flexor surface of the distal phalanx. Equine Vet Educ 2020;33(10).

76. Hoaglund E, Barrett M. Magnetic resonance imaging changes of the navicular bursa following navicular bursoscopy in seven horses. Equine Vet Educ; 2020.

77. Bladon BM, Giorio M. Correlation and prognostic value of abnormalities on MRI and navicular bursoscopy in horses with foot lameness. Vet Comp Orthop Traumatol 2018;31:A3651.

78. Smith M, Wright I. Endoscopic evaluation of the navicular bursa: observations, treatment and outcome in 92 cases with identified pathology. Equine Vet J 2012;44:339–45.
79. Humbach K, Gutierrez-Nibeyro S. Desmotomy of the accessory ligament of the deep digital flexor tendon for treatment of chronic deep digital flexor tendinopathy in three Quarter Horses. Equine Vet Educ 2018;30:538–44.
80. Gutierrez-Nibeyro S, Werpy N, White N, et al. Outcome of palmar/plantar digital neurectomy in horses with foot pain evaluated with magnetic resonance imaging: 50 cases (2005–2011). Equine Vet J 2015;47:160–4.

Moving?

Make sure your subscription moves with you!

To notify us of your new address, find your **Clinics Account Number** (located on your mailing label above your name), and contact customer service at:

Email: journalscustomerservice-usa@elsevier.com

800-654-2452 (subscribers in the U.S. & Canada)
314-447-8871 (subscribers outside of the U.S. & Canada)

Fax number: 314-447-8029

**Elsevier Health Sciences Division
Subscription Customer Service
3251 Riverport Lane
Maryland Heights, MO 63043**

*To ensure uninterrupted delivery of your subscription, please notify us at least 4 weeks in advance of move.

Printed and bound by CPI Group (UK) Ltd, Croydon, CR0 4YY

03/10/2024

01040470-0001